A Short Textbook of

ORAL RADIOLOGY

A Short Textbook of
ORAL RADIOLOGY

SECOND EDITION

C Anand Kumar BDS MDS

Senior Professor
Department of Oral Medicine and Radiology
AECS Maaruti College of Dental Sciences and Research Center
Bengaluru, Karnataka, India

Formerly

Professor and Head
Department of Oral Medicine and Radiology
PDM Dental College and Research Institute
Bahadurgarh, Haryana, India

Professor and Head
Department of Oral Medicine and Radiology
Kanti Devi Dental College and Hospital
Mathura, Uttar Pradesh, India

JAYPEE

JAYPEE BROTHERS MEDICAL PUBLISHERS

The Health Sciences Publisher

New Delhi | London

Jaypee Brothers Medical Publishers (P) Ltd.

Headquarters
EMCA House
23/23-B, Ansari Road, Daryaganj
New Delhi 110 002, India
Landline: +91-11-23272143,
+91-11-23272703
+91-11-23282021, +91-11-23245672
E-mail: jaypee@jaypeebrothers.com

Corporate Office
Jaypee Brothers Medical Publishers (P) Ltd.
4838/24, Ansari Road, Daryaganj
New Delhi 110 002, India
Phone: +91-11-43574357
Fax: +91-11-43574314
E-mail: jaypee@jaypeebrothers.com

Overseas Office
JP Medical Ltd.
83, Victoria Street, London
SW1H 0HW (UK)
Phone: +44-20 3170 8910
E-mail: info@jpmedpub.com

EU GPSR Authorised Representative
Logos Europe, 9 rue Nicolas Poussin
17000, La Rochelle, France
Phone: +33 (0) 6 67 93 73 78
E-mail: Contact@logoseurope.eu

Website: www.jaypeebrothers.com
Website: www.jaypeedigital.com

A Short Textbook of Oral Radiology

First Edition: 2004

Second Edition: 2018, Reprint: **2025**

ISBN: 978-93-5270-208-4

Printed in India

Dedicated to

My beloved

Students

Parents

Wife and Children

Preface to the Second Edition

After a gap of decade, the second edition is coming up; eventually, during this time, we have witnessed great advances in the field of diagnostic imaging. To keep abreast of new developments, the first edition has been revised thoroughly with new knowledge and technology.

In this edition, three new chapters on quality assurance, radiographic interpretation of dental caries and periodontal diseases have been included. Many chapters have been extensively rewritten and expanded to provide new emphasis on diagnostic radiology. New radiographic images are digitized with marking arrows over the lesions to explain radiographic features accurately. Detailed information is given on prevention and management of radiotherapy effects.

Interpretation of cysts and tumors chapters are revised and updated to present concepts so that students can update their knowledge to current scenario. The addition of radiographic images and illustrations provides valuable information on pathology of the diseases.

C Anand Kumar

Preface to the First Edition

The purpose of the book remains to give the dental provider an up-to-date, concise, factual reference work describing the basics in oral radiology.

In many instances, concepts are illustrated with a combination of radiographs and line drawings as well as tables, wherever applicable. There is extensive use of these aids to help the students understand more clearly and to clarify complex ideas.

The content is sufficiently detailed to satisfy the requirements of most undergraduate and postgraduate dental examinations. Some topics may have been inevitably omitted or sometimes oversimplified in condensing a very large and complex subject.

Apart from the use of bold heading and fonts of various sizes to clearly delineate subheadings from major headings, all of these format variations are designed to stimulate the students in the learning process, and give the students a feeling of comfort and ease in reading the book. The result I hope is a clear, logical and easily understandable text, that makes a contribution to the challenging task of teaching and learning dental radiology.

C Anand Kumar

Acknowledgments

I would like to express my gratitude to the many people who saw me through this book; to all those who provided support, talked things over, read, wrote, offered comments, allowed me to quote their remarks and assisted in the editing, proofreading and design.

I would like to thank the editorial staff at the M/s Jaypee Brothers Medical Publishers (P) Ltd, New Delhi, India, a special word of thanks goes to Shri Jitendar P Vij (Group Chairman) and Mr Ankit Vij (Group President), for enabling me to publish this book. Above all, I want to thank my parents, wife, sons, brothers, sisters and the rest of my family, who supported and encouraged me in spite of all the time it took me away from them. It was a long and difficult journey for them.

I am most thankful for the generous support from the department staff and well-wishers. Finally, I am grateful to our students, whose doubts and new things in their mind consistently discover new ways for me to improve each edition.

Last and not least, I beg forgiveness of all those who have been with me over the course of the years, and whose names I have failed to mention.

Contents

CHAPTER

1

Radiation Physics

The radiographs are considered as an adjunct in oral diagnosis and play a vital role in detecting, evaluating and even treated various lesions of the oral and para oral structures.

The radiographer must have thorough knowledge in interpretation of various normal and abnormal structures in the radiographs. For proper interpretation, radiographer can begin to understand X-radiation and its role in dentistry.

DEFINITIONS

Radiology: Radiology is a branch of medical science that deals with the study of radiation and its use, radioactive substances and other forms of radiant energy in the diagnosis and treatment of diseases.

Radiation: Radiation is a form of energy carried by waves or stream of particles, which transmit through space and matter.

X-radiation: X-radiation is a high energy radiation produced by the collision of a beam of electrons with a metal target in an X-ray tube.

X-ray: X-ray is a beam of energy that has the power to penetrate substances and record image shadows on photographic film.

Radiograph: Radiograph is an image on a film which is visible when viewed under transillumination, produced by the passage of X-rays through an object or body.

Radiography: It is the art and science of making radiographs by the exposure of films to X-rays.

HISTORY OF DENTAL RADIOLOGY

On the night of November 8, 1895, a tiny bit of fluorescence was noticed in laboratory by *Wilhelm Conrad Roentgen* and he called them as X-ray (unknown rays). He was a professor of physics at the physical institute of the Julius Maximilian University at Würzburg, subsequently he was awarded the first Nobel Prize in physics in 1901 **(Table 1.1)**.

Table 1.1: History of dental radiography

1895, November 8	Discovery of X-rays	Wilhelm Conrad Roentgen
1896, February	First dental radiograph	Otto Walkhoff
1896	First intraoral radiograph on live person	Edmund Kells
1898	Early announcement of danger of X-rays	William Herbert Rollins
1904	Introduction of bisecting technique	WA Price
1909	First course in radiography	HR Raper
1910	First dental X-ray laboratory	Franklin W McCormack
1913	First X-ray tube	WD Coolidge
1913	First dental X-ray films	Eastman Kodak Company
1923	First dental X-ray machine	Victor X-ray Corporation of Chicago
1925	Introduction of bitewing radiography	HR Raper
1947	Introduction of long cone technique	G Fitzgerald
1933	Principles of panoramic radiography	Numata
1978	Introduction of dental xeroradiography	
1981	Introduction of E-speed film	
1987	Intraoral digital radiography	

RADIATION PHYSICS

Atom is the fundamental unit of matter, consists of central nucleus made up of nuclear particles protons and neutrons surrounded by electrons in specific orbits or shells. An atom contains a maximum of seven orbits and they designated with the letters K, L, M, N, O, P and Q each located at a specific distance from the nucleus and representing different energy levels. The nucleus has a positive charge and an electron carries negative charge. Atom is electrically neutral when number of protons equal to number of electrons **(Fig. 1.1)**.

The number of protons and neutrons in an atom refer to the mass weight or atomic weight. The number of protons equals to the number of electrons determines the atomic number of the atom. Atoms differ from one another by its atomic weight and atomic number. Atoms are arranged in increasing atomic number on a chart.

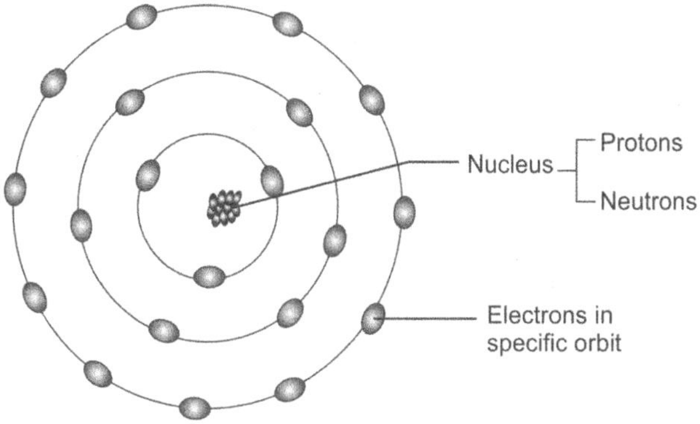

Fig. 1.1: Atom showing central nucleus and orbiting electrons

The electrostatic force of attraction between the positively charged nucleus (protons and neutrons) and negatively charged electrons maintains them in their orbits about the nucleus known as binding energy. Binding energy is determined by the distance between the nucleus and the orbital electrons. The strongest binding energy is found close to the nucleus in the k-shell, whereas outer shell electrons have a weak binding energy. Binding energies of electrons are measured in electron-volts (eV) or kilo electron-volts (keV). The energy required to remove an electron from its orbit must exceed the binding energy of the electron in that orbit. A greater amount of energy required to remove inner orbital electrons in contrast to the outer orbital electrons that required lesser energy.

For example, tungsten atom contains five orbits, the energy required to remove electrons from its inner orbit is 70 keV (70,000 eV) in contrast to the outer orbit that required 3 keV (3,000 eV).

IONIZATION

Atoms exist in either electrically neutral or in unbalanced state. A neutral atom contains an equal number of protons (positive charges) and electrons (negatively charges). Neutral atoms become unbalanced when externally force applied such as heating or collisions can cause loosening or gaining of electrons from the adjacent atom. If the atom gains an electron, it has more electrons than protons and therefore a negative charge. Similarly atom loses electron has more protons and less electrons become positive charge. An atom gains or loses electron and becomes electrically unbalanced known as ion.

Ionization is the process of converting an atom into ions. When electrically neutral atom loses an electron, it becomes a positive ion and the free electron a negative ion. Ionization also produced by addition of an electrically neutral atom resulting in a negative ion. Note that protons do not participate in this process. Electrons can be removed from an atom by various means such as heating, collisions with high energy X-rays.

RADIATION

Types of Radiation

Radiation is the transmission of energy through space and matter. Radiation can be classified into two groups:

1. Particulate radiation
2. Electromagnetic radiation

Particulate Radiation

Particulate radiations are tiny particles of matter that possess mass and moving at high velocity. For example, alpha particles, beta particles and cathode rays.

Alpha particles are helium nuclei consisting of two protons and two neutrons result from the radioactive decay of elements. Alpha particles densely ionize matter (penetrate tissue of short length) because of their high charge, low velocity and heavy mass.

Beta particles are electrons emitted by radioactive nuclei. Because of their higher velocity, light mass and lower charge they are able to penetrate matter to a greater depth than the alpha particles.

Cathode rays are streams of high speed electrons that produced in an X-ray tube.

Electromagnetic Radiation

Electromagnetic radiation is the movement of wave like energy through space or matter as a combination of electric and magnetic fields **(Fig. 1.2)**. It is generated when the velocity of an electrically charged particle is altered, e.g. gamma-rays, X-rays, ultraviolet rays, visible light, infrared radiation (heat), television, radar and microwaves.

The electromagnetic radiation can be classified depending on their energy into:

- Ionizing
- Nonionizing

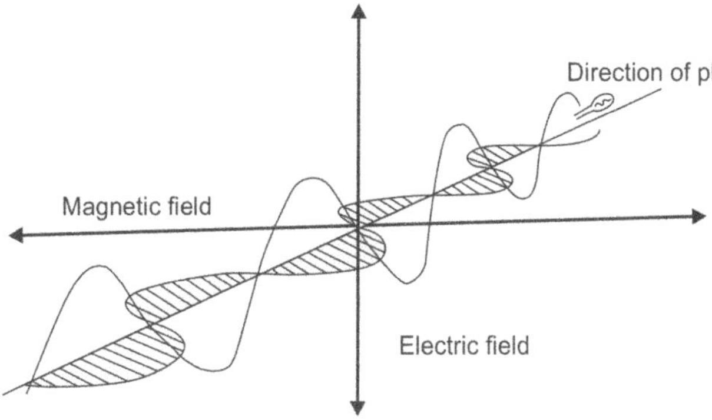

Fig. 1.2: Electromagnetic radiation

Ionizing: If there is sufficient energy associated with the radiation to remove orbital electrons from the atoms in the irradiated matter (ionization), the radiation is said to be ionizing radiation (e.g. cosmic rays, γ-rays and X-rays).

Nonionizing: Those rays, which are not able to remove electrons from the atom are said to be nonionizing radiation (e.g. radiowaves, microwaves, infrared and ultraviolet rays).

Electromagnetic radiations are move through space and matter as both particle and a wave.

In particle concept, radiations are move through space as a bundle of energy called as photons or quanta at the speed of light.

In wave concept, electromagnetic radiations are travel in waves with a specific frequency at the speed of light.

Wavelength can be defined as the distance between the crest of the two waves **(Fig. 1.3)**. Wavelength determines the energy and penetrating power of the radiation, the shorter the distance between the crests, the shorter the wavelength and high penetrating power and vice versa. Wavelength is measured in nanometers.

Frequency is described as the numbers of wavelengths that pass at given point in a certain amount of time. Wavelengths and frequency are inversely proportional, if frequency is high wavelength is short and vice versa **(Fig. 1.4)**. The amount of energy of an electromagnetic radiation depends on the wavelength and frequency. Low energy electromagnetic radiations (e.g. radiowaves and microwaves) have longer wavelength and low frequency in contrast to high energy radiations such as X-rays and γ-rays, have short wavelength and high frequency **(Table 1.2)**.

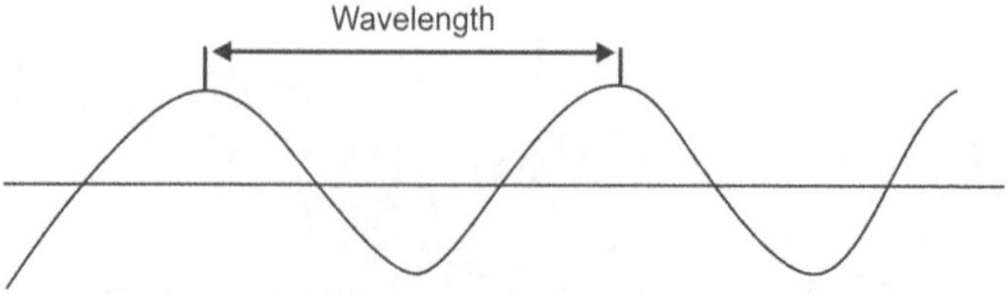

Fig. 1.3: Wavelength (Distance between the two crests)

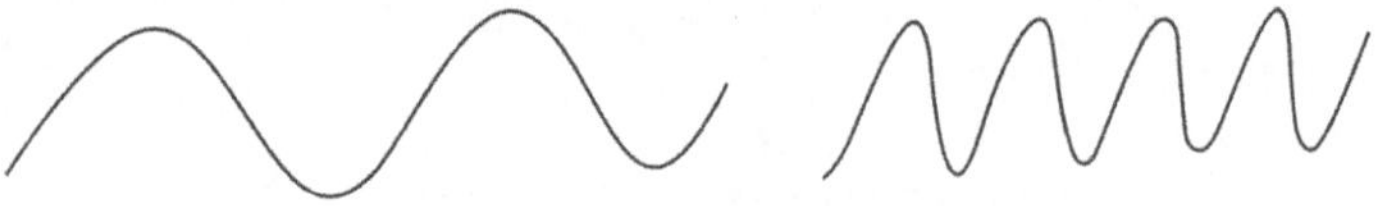

Fig. 1.4: Relation between wavelength and frequency

Table 1.2: Electromagnetic radiation as it relates to wavelength and energy

Short wavelength/higher energy	*Longer wavelength/lower energy*
γ-rays	UV light
X-rays	Visible light
	Infrared
	Radar
	Microwaves
	Television
	Radiowaves
	Electric waves

X-RAY MACHINE

X-ray machine contains X-ray tube and the power supply.

X-ray Tube

It is also called *Coolidge tube* because it follows the design of WC Coolidge, who introduced in 1913. The X-ray tube is a glass vacuum tube from which all of the air has been expelled. The basic apparatus for generating X-rays by X-ray tube, composed **(Fig. 1.5)**.

- Cathode
- Anode

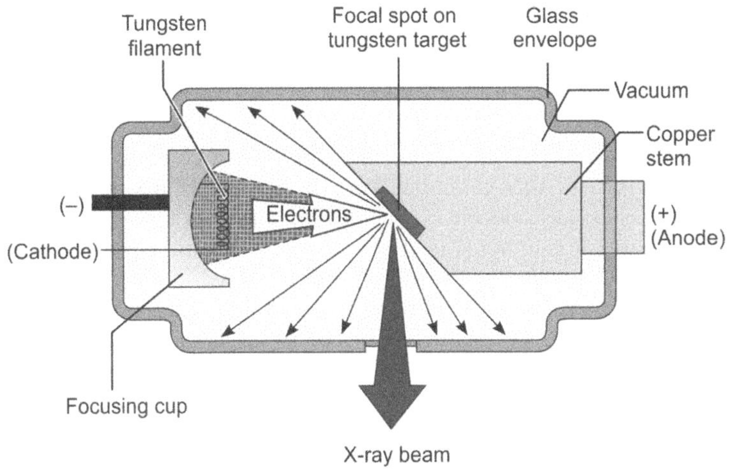

Fig. 1.5: Schematic diagram of X-ray tube

Cathode and anode are encased within an evacuated glass envelope or tube. Electrical power supply is necessary to accelerating the electrons.

Cathode

It is composed of two parts:

1. Filament
2. Focusing cup

Filament is the source of electrons within the X-ray tube, made up of tungsten wire, connected to electric current. When filament is heated it emits the electrons. A milliampere (mA) control provides for fine adjustment of voltage across the filament and in turn the flow of heating current through it, there by it controls the quantity (number) of electrons.

Focusing cup is a negatively charged concave reflector cup made up of molybdenum which focuses the electrons emitted by filament into a narrow beam directed at a focal spot an anode. Which attracts negatively charged electrons. To facilitate the movement of these high-speed electrons the X-ray tube is evacuated so as to avoid collision of moving electrons with air molecules, which reduces their speed and burnout of the filament due to oxidation.

Anode

Anode is composed of:
- *Tungsten target*
- *Copper stem.*

Tungsten target: The purpose of the target is to convert the kinetic energy of the electrons generated from the filament into X-ray photons. Tungsten is usually selected as the target material because of:
- High atomic number (74) (higher the atomic number denser is the metal required to stop the high speed electrons).
- High melting point (To with stand the lot of heat generated during collisions of high velocity electrons to the target metal).
- Low vapor pressure at the high working temperature of an X-ray tube (Since electron beams are directed to a small area of the target, some of the atoms may reach the vapor state causing blisters on the metal target which reduces the life of the target).

Copper stem: The target is embedded in a large block of copper. Copper is a good thermal conductor, which dissipates the heat generated when sudden stopping of high voltage electrons at the target. The sharpness of radiographic image increases as the focal spot decreases. The focal spot is the area on the target on to which the focusing cups directs the electrons from the filament.

Power Supply

To understand how the X-ray tube functions and X-rays are produced, the dental radiographer must understand some aspects of an electrical current, electrical circuit and transformer.

Electrical current: Electrical current is the movement of electrons through conductor. Two types of current are:
1. Direct current (DC)
2. Alternating current (AC).

Direct current describes a current in which the electrons flow in one direction through the conductor. But in alternating current, electrons flow in two opposite directions.

In *alternating current* high voltage applied between the cathode and anode. When electrons strike the focal spot of the target, some of their energy converts to X-ray photons. Because of the AC current (60 cycles per second), the polarity of the AC reversed after half of the cycle (negative cycle), the filament becomes positive and the target becomes negative. At these time no movement of electrons across the tube; hence

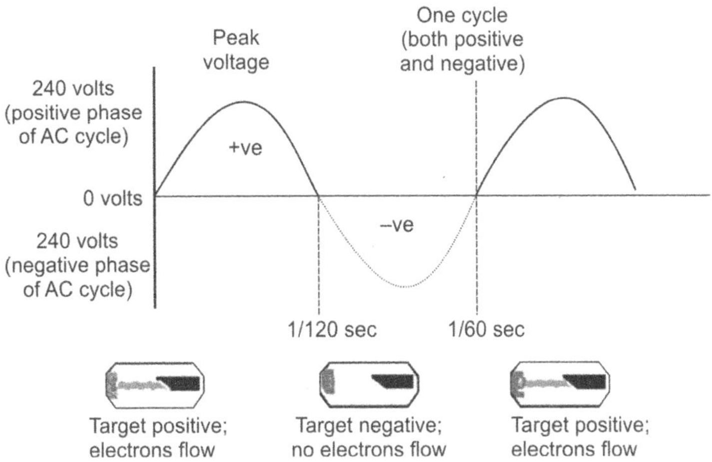

Fig. 1.6: Alternating current during positive cycle results in X-ray production, but during negative cycle, no X-ray production occurs

no X-rays are generated during this negative half of the AC cycle. This type of power supply circuit limits the production of X-rays to half and is called *self rectification* or *half-wave rectification* **(Fig. 1.6)**.

During inverse voltage (negative half of the cycle during which cathode become anode and vice versa), X-ray tube target (anode) started emitting electrons towards the filament (cathode) results in overheating and melting of the filament and also damage to the glass envelope. This can be prevented automatically by the process of self or half wave rectification adopted in the X-ray machine itself.

Modern dental X-ray machines, which replaces the conventional 60 cycle AC high voltage current of the X-ray tube with a high frequency DC power supply. In high frequency DC power supply, current flows in one direction (i.e., from cathode to anode), which results in production of high mean energy of the X-ray photons than the conventional half wave rectified machine operated at the same voltage, which reduced the amount of low energy X-ray photons thereby reduce in the patient exposure to radiation **(Fig. 1.7)**.

Electrical circuits: Two electrical circuits are used in the production of X-rays:

1. Low voltage or filament circuit
2. High voltage circuit.

The low voltage filament circuit uses 7–10 volts to heat the X-ray tube filament and tube current flows from the filament to the anode and then

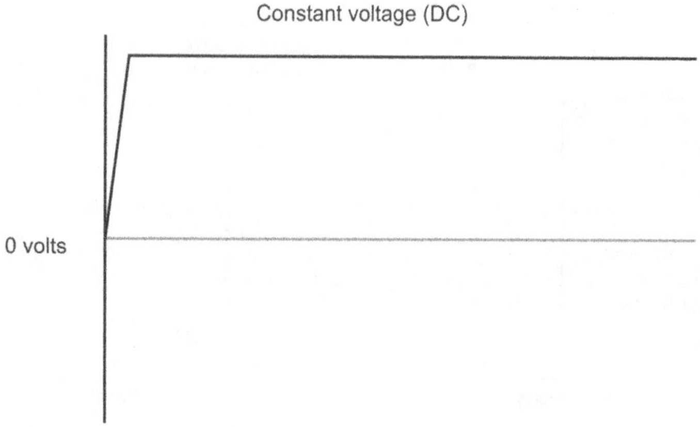

Fig. 1.7: DC current shows the constant voltage applied across the X-ray tube

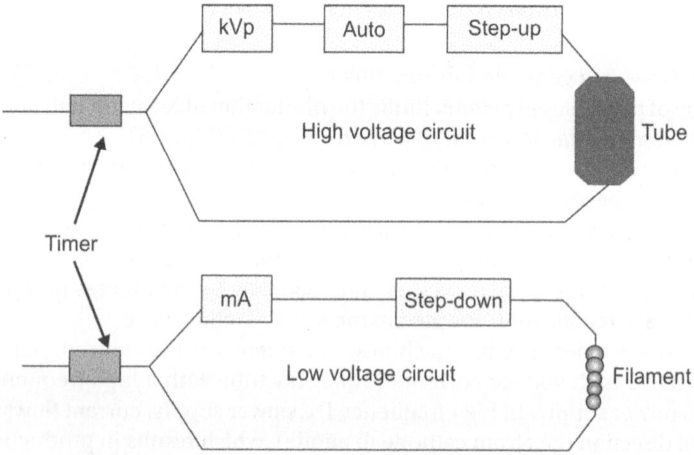

Fig. 1.8: High voltage circuit regulated by step-up and kVp. Low voltage circuit by mA and step-down transformer

back to the filament and is controlled by the milliampere settings (mA) and step-down transformer **(Fig. 1.8)**.

The high voltage circuit uses 60,000 to 1,00,000 volts (60–100 kV) applied across the tube to accelerate the electrons towards the anode target to generate the X-rays and is controlled by kilovoltage settings (kVp), step-up and auto-transformer **(Fig. 1.8)**.

Transformers

A transformer is a device that is used to either increase or decrease the line voltage (220 volts) in an electrical circuit. Three types of transformers are used in dental X-ray tube:

- Step-down transformer,
- Step-up transformer, and
- Autotransformer.

Step down transformer is used in filament circuit to decrease the voltage from incoming 220 volts to 7–10 volts to heats up the filament in cathode.

Step-up transformers are required to increase the 220 line volts into 60,000–1,00,000 volts in high voltage circuit to accelerate the electrons towards the target. Auto transformer serves as a voltage compensator that corrects for minor voltage fluctuations.

PRODUCTION OF X-RAYS

When the X-ray machine turned on, current flow into the filament circuit, which contains step down transformer to reduce the usual voltage of 220 into 7–10 volts required to heat the tungsten filament. When filament heated up which releases the electrons (Thermionic emission) and an electron cloud forms around the filament. When the exposure button is pressed, current flow into the step-up transformer where 220 line volts change into 60–100 kV required to accelerate the electrons move towards the anode target. When the sudden stopping of these high energy electrons at the focal spot of a target occur, these high energy electrons are converted into X-rays (1%) and generates lot of heat (99%). X-ray beam comes out through the small window created in the X-ray tube and heat is carried away through the copper at anode and also absorbed by the oil, which circulates in the glass envelope of X-ray machine.

The kinetic energy of electrons in the tube, converted into X-ray photons at the focal spot of an X-ray tube by two mechanisms:

1. Bremsstrahlung radiation
2. Characteristic radiation

Bremsstrahlung Radiation

Most of the X-rays (70%) are produced by Bremsstrahlung radiation only. When the high speed electrons (high speed electrons are produced by accelerating electrons to a high velocity by the high voltage applied across the gap between the filament and target of X-ray tube) hits the nucleus of a target atom, all of its kinetic energy will be converted into

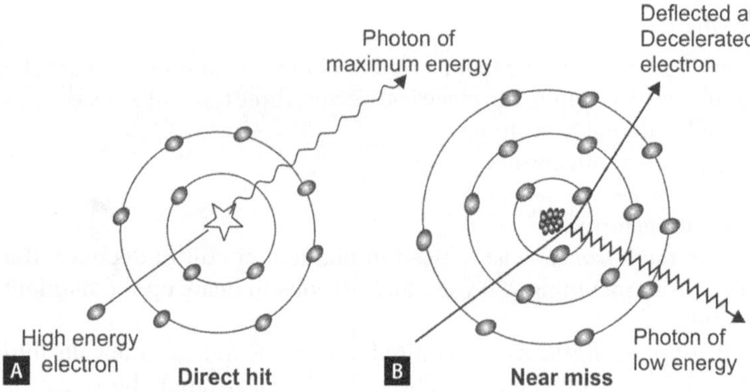

Figs 1.9A and B: Bremsstrahlung radiation is produced by the direct hit of electrons on the nucleus in the target (A) or by the near miss (B)

a single X-ray photon of maximal energy. The energy of the resultant photon is equal to the energy of the electron.

Most of the high-speed electrons have pass just near to the nucleus causing negatively charged electrons are attracted toward the positively charged nucleus and loses some of its kinetic energy results in electron being deflected and decelerated. This energy is given off in the form of low energy photon **(Figs 1.9A and B)**.

Characteristic Radiation

Characteristic radiation occurs when a high-energy electron hits the target atom, which ejects the electron from inner orbit, creating vacancy. This inner vacancy is quickly filled with electron from outer orbit. When the displaced electron is replaced by the outer shell electron, a photon is emitted with energy equivalent to difference in the energy level of two orbits **(Figs 1.10A to D)**. It is only a minor source of radiation from an X-ray tube.

PROPERTIES OF X-RAYS

Properties of X-ray are divided into:

- General properties
- Diagnostic properties
- Biologic properties
- Miscellaneous

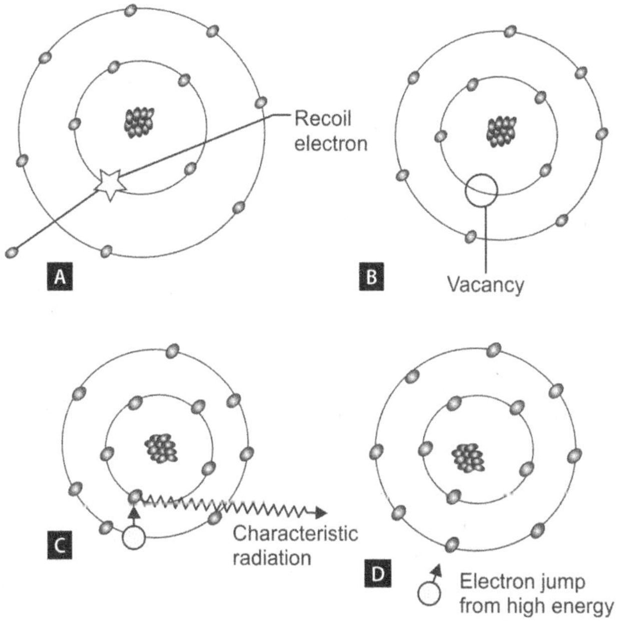

Figs 1.10A to D: Characteristic radiation. (A) Incident electron hit the inner orbital electron results in ejection of electron; (B) Vacancy created in the orbit; (C) This vacancy is filled by outer orbital electron and the photon is emitted; (D) Similar process of jumping of electrons from the other orbit

General Properties

- X-rays are travel in straight lines and can be deflected or scattered.
- Speed of the X-ray is equal to the speed of the light.
- X-rays are invisible.
- Shorter wavelength X-ray possess greater energy with greater penetration power.
- X-ray beam is made up of millions of photons of different energies
- Electric or magnetic field cannot deflect X-rays.
- They are the electromagnetic radiation.
- Intensity of X-rays obeys the inverse square law (intensity inversely proportional to the distance).
- X-rays cannot be focused to a point and always diverge from a point.

Diagnostic Properties

- X-rays can affect film emulsion to produce a visual image.
- X-rays are fluorescing the phosphor salts.

- It can neutralize electric charges on selenium coated plates (in Xero radiography)
- It can activate on charge coupled device (CCD) used in digital radiography.

Biologic Properties

X-rays are capable of producing ionization and thus causing biological damage in living tissue.

Miscellaneous

It can produce some color changes in certain materials (Doppler system).

FACTORS CONTROLLING X-RAY BEAM

The X-ray beam emitted from the X-ray tube may be modified to suit the requirements of the application.

This may be accomplished by:

- Altering the X-ray tube operation (kVp, mA and exposure time).
- Manipulation of the X-ray beam (filtration, collimation and target to film distance).
- Controlling the interactions between the X-ray beam and the object (Grids).

Tube voltage (kVp): Voltage is a measurement of electrical force between the two opposite charges. Voltage is measured in volts or kilovolts. Voltage meter on the control panel measures the X-ray tube voltage. Dental radiography requires the use of 65–100 kV.

The use less than 65 kV produce less penetrating X-ray beam with less energy and longer wavelengths that does not have adequate energy to penetrate into the dental tissues for diagnostic needs of the patients. Where as more than 100 kV produce greater energy and shorter wavelengths which results in over penetration into the tissues.

Kilovoltage peak (kVp) is a maximum or peak voltage. The kVp regulates the speed and energy of the electrons between cathode and anode and determines the penetrating energy of the X-ray beam.

When kVp is increased, voltage potential between the cathode and the anode increased which in-turn results in increase in the energy of each electron strikes the target which leads to conversion of electron energy into X-ray photons, and thus increase in:

- Quality (energy) of photons
- Mean energy of the photons
- Maximum energy of photons.

Effect of Kilovoltage Peak on Density and Contrast

Density means overall darkening or blackening of a film. Density of the radiograph can be altered by the adjustment in kilovoltage peak. When the kilovoltage peak is increased while other exposure factors (Milliamperage, exposure time) remain constant, the resultant film exhibits an increased density and appears dark radiograph. If kilovoltage peak is decreased, the resultant film exhibits a decreased density and appears light radiograph **(Table 1.3)**.

Contrast refers to the difference in densities between various regions on the film so that it can able to differentiate between the light and dark areas in the radiograph. An adjustment in kilovoltage peak results in a change in the contrast of the radiograph. If the kilovoltage is increased, the resultant image appears low contrast (many shades of gray instead of light and dark areas). A film with low contrast is useful for the detection of periodontal and periapical diseases. When the kilovoltage peak decreased, the image appears high contrast (few shades of gray and many white and dark areas). High contrast film is useful in detection and progression of dental caries **(Table 1.3)**.

Tube current (mA): The ampere is a unit of measurement of the number of electrons or current flowing through the cathode. Milliamperage regulates the temperature of the cathode filament. A higher milliampere setting increases the temperature of the cathode filament and consequently increases the number of electrons at the cathode. When more number of electrons strikes the target, greater number (quantity) of X-ray photons are produced. The quantity (number) of photons produced by the X-ray tube is directly related to tube current. Thus increase in the tube current will produce more number of photons. In dental radiography 7–15 milliamperage is required.

An increase in milliamperage increases the overall density of the radiograph and results in a darker image. Conversely, a decrease in milliamperage decreases the density of the radiograph and results in a lighter image.

Milliamperage and exposure time are inversely related, when milliamperage is increased, the exposure time must be decreased and

Table 1.3: Effect of kilovoltage on density and contrast

	Density	*Contrast*
Increased kVp	Increased density (Dark radiograph)	Low (Long gray scale)
Decreased kVp	Decreased density (Light radiograph)	High (Short gray scale)

conversely, when milliamperage is decreased, the exposure time must be increased to maintain the diagnostic density of a radiograph.

Exposure time: A timer is installed into the high voltage circuit to control the duration of the X-ray exposure. The timer controls the length of time that high voltage is applied to the tube and therefore the time during which current flows to the filament and X-rays are produced. In X-ray machine, timers are calibrated in seconds or fractions of seconds. If exposure time is increased, while the mA and kVp held constant, number of photons generated is doubled, but the photon energies is unchanged. Thus, the effect of changing exposure time is simply to control the quantity of the photons.

Milliampere-seconds (mAs): A combination of milliampere and exposure time. When milliamperage increased, the exposure time must be decreased and vice versa. Select the higher milliamperage X-ray machine when less exposure time is required in the dental radiography.

Filtration: Discussed in Chapter 3.

Collimation: Discussed in Chapter 3.

Target to film distance: Inverse square law states that intensity of the X-ray beam is inversely proportional to the square of the distance from the source of radiation.

Intensity of the X-ray beam diminishes as distance increased because the X-ray beam is divergent, i.e. it spreads out as it moves from the source and numbers of photons are decreased as it moves away from the source. Thus to get the high contrast of the image in case of long cone technique where X-ray and the object are in a long distance to increase the kVp and mA to maintain the high intensity of the X-ray beam.

Grids: Discussed in Chapter 7.

X-RAY INTERACTIONS WITH MATTER

When X-rays are interact with matter, X-ray photons are attenuated by:

- Absorption (conversion of their energy into kinetic energy of absorber electrons)
- Scattering of X-ray photons out of the absorber as a result of interaction with the orbital electrons of component atom **(Figs 1.11A to C)**.

There are three mechanisms by which absorption and scattering processes take place:

1. Coherent scattering
2. Photoelectric effect
3. Compton effect

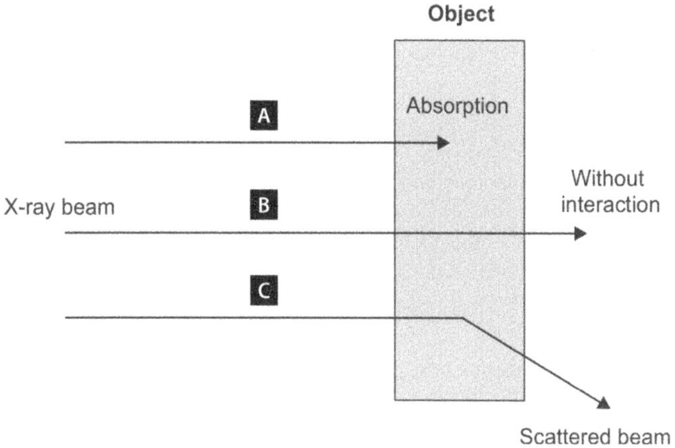

Figs 1.11A to C: Three types of X-ray interaction. (A) Beam indicates absorption within the object itself; (B) Refers to X-ray beam pass out of the object without any interactions. (C) X-ray beam scattered out of the object as a result of interaction with the orbital electrons of object

Coherent Scattering

When a low energy X-ray photon passes near an atom of outer electron (having low binding energy) it may not be absorbed, but scattered without a loss of energy. This process is known as coherent scattering.

The incident photon interacts with the electron by causing it to vibrate momentarily. The incident photon then ceases to exist. The vibration then causes the electron to radiate energy in the form of another X-ray photon of the same frequency and energy as the incident beam **(Fig. 1.12)**. *This type of interaction accounts only for 8% of the total number of interactions in a dental radiography.* In diagnostic radiology, the effect of coherent scattering is negligible in producing film fog in comparison with the Compton effect.

Photoelectric Effect

Photoelectric absorption occurs when incident photon strikes the inner orbital electron and gives up all its energy, and it ejected from the atom as photoelectron. Electron vacancy in inner orbit is filled by electron from higher energy level, this causes emission of characteristic radiation and this vacancy filled by electrons of other orbit thus completing energy exchange. The ejected electrons travel only a short distance in the absorber before they dissipate all their energy. All of the energy of incident photons that undergo photoelectric interaction is deposited in

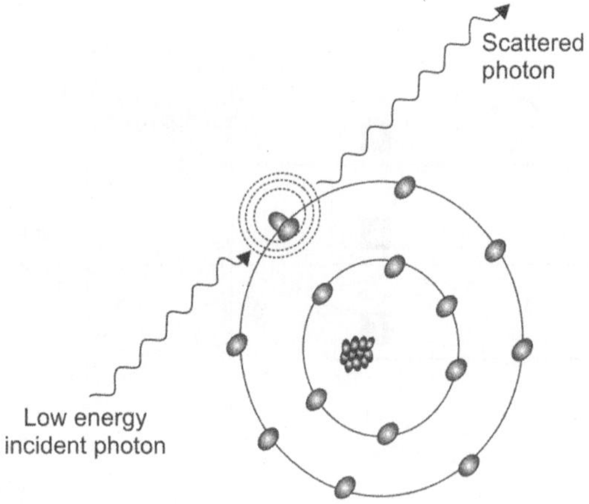

Fig. 1.12: Scattered photon results when low energy incident photon interacts with the outer orbital electron, causing it to vibrate momentarily. After this, scattered photon is emitted at different angle than incident photon

the absorber **(Figs 1.13A to D)**. This is good for the dentist because there is no scattered radiation, but bad for the patient because for increased radiation absorption. *This type of interaction accounts 30%.*

Compton Effect

Compton effect occurs when a photon interacts with a outer orbital electron (free electron).

In this interaction, the incident photon collides with an outer electron, resulting in a scattered photon of lower energy then incident photon and a recoil electron ejected from target atom **(Fig. 1.14)**. In dental radiograph, *Compton interactions undergo 62%.* During a dental X-ray exposure, 30% of the scattered X-ray photons exit the patient's head. This is advantageous to the patient because some of the incident photon escapes the tissue, but it is disadvantageous to the dentist because it may cause film fog.

DOSIMETRY

Dosimetry is the measurement of quantity of radiation exposure or amount of energy absorbed per unit mass at an interest site (dose).

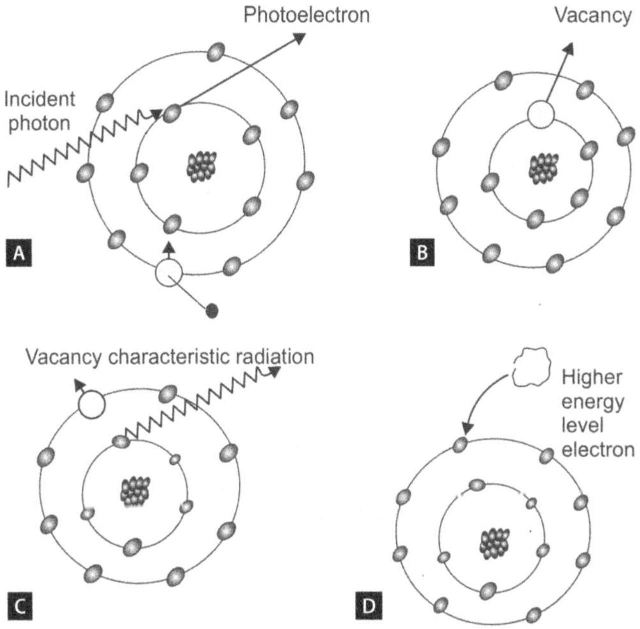

Figs 1.13A to D: (A) Photoelectric absorption occurs when incident photon gives up all its energy to inner electron causing ejection of electron as a photoelectron; (B) Vacancy in inner orbit occurs. (C) Vacancy is filled by outer orbital electron and emits characteristic radiation. (D) Process of filling electron vacancy continues till the completion of energy exchange

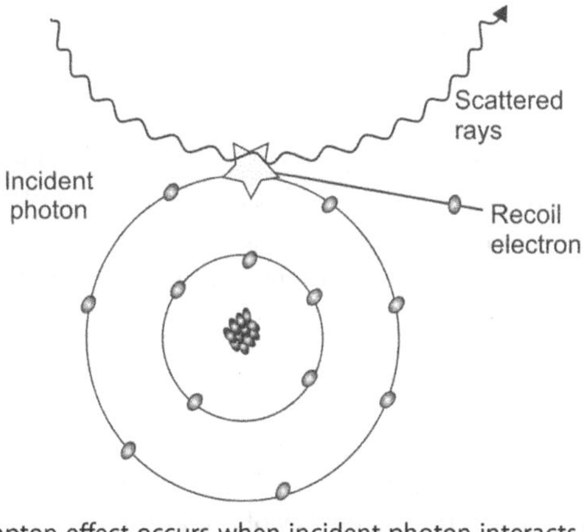

Fig. 1.14: Compton effect occurs when incident photon interacts with the outer orbital electron results in scattered photon of low energy and ejection of recoil electron

A variety of techniques are available for such measurements based on the ability of radiation to cause ionization in air under standard conditions of temperature and pressure.

- Ionization chambers
- Film badges
- Thermoluminescent dosimeters

Ionization Chambers

It can be described as pair of collecting plates with an opposite charge and separated by a standard volume of air. The plates are connected to an electrometer, which is capable of measures small electric charge. When an X-ray beam is directed through the air in the chamber causes generation of ions by interaction of X-ray beam with air molecules. The positive and negative ions are attracted by plates cause partial discharge and it is measured by magnitude of the drop in potential between the collecting plates.

Advantages

- Most accurate method of measuring radiation dose.
- Direct read-out gives immediate information.

Disadvantages

- They give no permanent record of exposure.
- No indication of the type of radiation.
- They are not very sensitive to low energy radiation.

Film Badges

X-ray film may be used to monitor radiation exposure to the dental radiographer. The film is usually worn in metallic badges. The film is subsequently processed and measures the degree of darkening. It must be comparison with films exposed to known amounts of radiation results in darkening. Such film badges are often used to monitor the degree of exposure to individuals.

Advantages

- It provides a permanent record of exposure.
- May be checked and reassessed at a later date.
- Can measure the type and energy of radiation.
- Simple and inexpensive.

Disadvantages

- No immediate indication of exposure
- Give errors while processing.

Thermoluminescent Dosimeters

Certain crystals such as lithium fluoride have a special property to absorb radiation energy and subsequently release it as a visible light on heating the crystals. The total visible light emitted by the crystals is proportional to the energy absorbed by the crystals.

Advantages

- Lithium fluoride crystals are reusable.
- Suitable for wide variety of dose measurements
- Measurements are rapidly produced and it is accurate.

Disadvantages

- Results cannot be checked or reassessed.
- Relatively expensive.

UNITS OF MEASUREMENT

- *Exposure:* Exposure is a measure of quantity of radiation and it is measured by
  Traditional unit: Roentgen
  SI unit: Coulomb/kg
- *Absorbed dose:* Is a measure of the energy imparted by any type of ionizing radiation to a mass of any type of matter.
  Traditional unit: Gray
  SI unit: Rad
- *Dose equivalent:* It is the basic unit of radiation protection.
  Traditional unit: Rem (Rad equivalent mammal)
  SI unit: Sievert (Sv)
- *Radioactivity:* It is the decay rate of a sample of radioactive material.
  Traditional unit: Becquerel
  SI unit: Curie

CHAPTER 2

Radiation Biology

BIOLOGICAL EFFECTS AND RISKS ASSOCIATED WITH X-RAYS

Radiation biology is the study of the effects of ionizing radiation on living systems. Initial changes are modification of biologic molecules may result in alterations in cells and organs that may persist for hours, decades, and possibly even for generations; such functional changes may result in death of the cells or organs.

The primary actions of radiation on living systems are of two types:
1. Direct effects
2. Indirect effects

Direct Effects

When the energy of photon is transferred directly to biological molecules the effect is termed direct effect which involves in three steps:
1. Absorption of energy by the biological molecule.
2. Transfer of energy between unstable intermediate molecules.
3. Formation of unstable free radicals.

(Free radical means molecules or atoms have unpaired electron in the valence shell and they are extremely reactive and have very short life, quickly reforming into stable damaged molecules by crosslinking).

Approximately 1/3rd of biologic effects of X-ray result from direct effects.

Indirect Effects

When the photon absorbed by water in a biological system and the water molecules are ionized, they form free radicals that react with biologic molecules and produce changes in the molecules. About two-thirds of radiation-induced biologic damage result from indirect effects.

Water is the predominant molecule in biologic systems (about 70%); it frequently participates in the interactions between X-rays photons and the biologic molecules of an organism. The hydrogen and hydroxyl free radical present in the water interacts with organic molecule result in the formation of organic-free radicals. Organic-free radicals are unstable, and transform into stable altered molecules. These altered molecules have different chemical and biologic properties. The hydroxyl (OH) free radicals combine to form toxins (e.g. H_2O_2), which cause cellular dysfunction and biologic damage.

CHANGES IN BIOLOGIC MOLECULES

Nucleic Acids

Cellular function is primarily determined by nucleic acids. If damage to the DNA molecules results in cell death after radiation exposure.

The following are changes in DNA:

- Change in a base.
- Disruption of hydrogen bonds between DNA strands
- Breakage of one or more DNA strands.
- Crosslinking of DNA strands with in the helix, to other DNA strands or to protein.

Proteins

- Breakage of hydrogen or disulfide bonds leads to denaturation of proteins.
- Intermolecular and intramolecular crosslinking.

RADIATION EFFECTS AT THE CELLULAR LEVEL

Initially, molecular changes are produced within a fraction of second after exposure, cellular changes resulting from moderate exposures usually required a minimum of hours to become apparent and manifest as structural and functional changes in cellular organelles later cell death may occur.

Nucleus

Nucleus is more radiosensitive than the cytoplasm, especially in dividing cells. DNA structures are sensitive site in the nucleus.

Chromosome Aberrations

Chromosome serves as markers for radiation injury. If radiation exposure occurs after DNA synthesis, only one arm of the affected chromosome is broken (chromatid aberration).

If radiation occurs before DNA synthesis, the damage manifests as a break in both arms (chromosome aberration) **(Figs 2.1A and B)**.

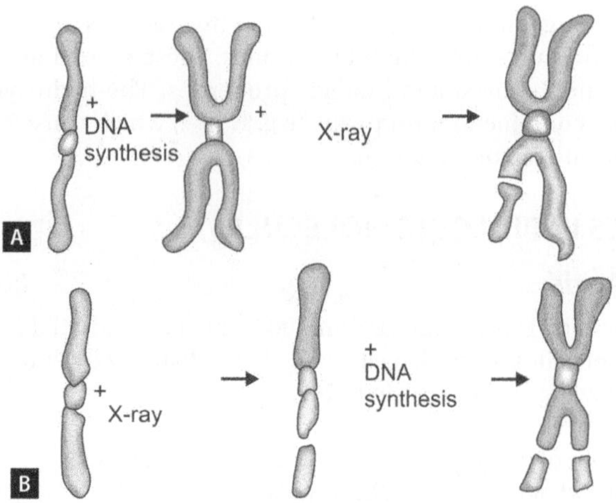

Figs 2.1A and B: Chromosome aberrations. (A) Radiation occurs after DNA synthesis causes defect in one arm of chromosome. (B) Both arms are defective when radiation occurs before DNA synthesis

Such radiation-induced aberrations may result in unequal distribution of chromatin material to daughter cells. Chromosome aberrations have been detected in peripheral blood lymphocytes of patient.

Cytoplasm

Mitochondria show increased permeability, swelling and disorganization of the internal cristae.

RADIATION EFFECTS AT THE TISSUE AND ORGAN LEVEL

Large number of cells death leads to affected organ display a clinical result. The severity of this change depends on the dose of radiation. There are two types of radiation effects on tissue and organ levels.
1. Nonstochastic effects
2. Stochastic effects

Nonstochastic Effects

Definitely or specific damaging effects to the body of the person exposed to the high dose of radiation. The severity of the effects is directly proportional to the dose received.

For example, reddening of skin, and cataract formation.

Stochastic Effects

The chances or probability of radiation effects may or may not be affecting the person. For example, leukemia and certain tumors.

These radiation effects are classified into:

- Short-term effects
- Long-term effects

Short-term Effects

Short-term effects of radiation on a tissue are depends primarily by the sensitivity of its cells. If continuously proliferating tissues (e.g. bone marrow, oral mucous membrane) are irradiated, more radiation injury to the cells. The extent of cells loss depends on proliferative rate of the cells.

If less proliferative rate or never dividing cells are irradiated (e.g. muscle), then demonstrate little or no radiation induced effects over the short term. **Table 2.1** shows the radiosensitivity of different organs.

Long-term Effects

The long-term effects of radiation on tissues and organs depend primarily on the extent of damage to the fine vasculature. Irradiation to the capillary causes swelling, degeneration and necrosis, which results in increased capillary permeability and initiate slow progressive fibrosis around the vessels leads to premature narrowing and obliteration of vascular lumens, which impairs the transport of oxygen, nutrients and waste products and results in death of cells. The net result is progressive fibroatrophy of the irradiated tissue.

Table 2.1: Radiosensitivity of various organs

High	*Intermediate*	*Low*
• Lymphoid organs	• Fine vasculature	• Optic lens
• Bone marrow	• Growing cartilage	• Mature erythrocytes
• Testes	• Growing bone	• Muscle cells
• Intestines	• Salivary glands	• Neurons
• Mucous membranes	• Lungs	
	• Kidney	
	• Liver	

MODIFYING FACTORS FOR RADIATION INJURY

The response of cells to radiation depends on:

- Variations in exposure parameters (dose and dose rate)
- The environment of the cells (oxygen and linear energy transfer)

Dose: The severity of damage in irradiated tissues or organs depends on the amount of radiation received. All the individuals receiving doses above the threshold level show damage to the tissues.

Dose rate: Dose rate indicates rate of exposure, e.g. total dose of 5 Gy may be given at a high dose rate (5 Gy/min) or a low dose rates (5 mGy/min). Exposure of tissue to a given dose at a high dose rate causes more damage than exposure to the same total dose given at a lower dose rate. When tissues are exposed at lower dose rates, a greater opportunity exists for repair of damage, thereby resulting in less tissue net damage.

Oxygen: The resistant of tissues to the irradiation depends on oxygen level in it. The presence of oxygen increases the cells sensitivity to radiation. If more oxygen level causes the tissue to become less resistance to the irradiation and vice versa.

Linear energy transfer: High linear energy transfer caused more biological effect than low linear energy transfer, e.g. alpha particles are high LET radiation causes more damaging biologic systems because of their high ionization than X-rays.

RADIATION EFFECTS ON THE ORAL CAVITY

Oral Mucous Membrane

During Irradiation

- *Mucositis:* Oral mucous membranes show areas of redness and inflammation.
- *Desquamated epithelial layer:* Mucous membranes begin to break-down, with the formation of a white to yellow pseudomembrane.
- *Severe mucositis:* Develops as irradiation continues results in difficult to intake of food.
- *Infection:* Infection of the oral cavity develops due to bad oral hygiene.
- Secondary infection by *Candida albicans.*

After Irradiation

- Mucosa begins to heal rapidly by about 2 months.
- Later day's mucosa becomes atrophic, thin and avascular; atrophy develops due to obliteration of the fine vasculature and fibrosis of the connective tissue.
- Ulcer results from a denture sore, radiation necrosis or tumor recurrence.

Treatment of radiation mucositis

- Maintaining good oral hygiene
- Oral rinses with saline, bicarbonate, dilute hydrogen peroxide and water.
- Lips applied with water-based lubricants and lanolin.
- Coating agents used as oral rinses such as milk of magnesia, liquid amphogel, cellulose and sucralfate.
- Topical anesthetics can be used such as lignocaine, dyclonine, benzocaine and diphenhydramine.
- Analgesics such as benzydamine hydrochloride used effectively to relieve the pain from mucositis.
- Infections can be controlled by chlorhexidine and systemic antimicrobials.
- Antifungal drugs such as nystatin, amphotericin B, ketoconazole 200 mg and 150 mg of fluconazole.

Taste Buds

Taste buds are sensitive to radiation and causing:

- Degeneration of taste buds
- Loss of taste sensation, bitter and acid flavors is more severely affected when posterior 2/3rd of tongue irradiated. Anterior 1/3rd of tongue irradiated causes loss of salt and sweet sensation. Recovery of taste buds requires 60–120 days after irradiation.

Salivary Glands

Parotid glands are more sensitive than the submandibular and sublingual glands.

- Progressive loss of salivary secretion
- *Xerostomia:* Dryness of mouth.
- Swallowing is difficult and painful because the residual saliva loses its normal lubricating properties.

- pH and buffering capacity of saliva falls down.
- Histologically, acute inflammatory response may occur soon after the initiation of therapy. Progressive fibrosis, adiposis, loss of fine vasculature and degeneration of parenchyma results in xerostomia.
- Salivary changes influence on the oral microflora. Leading to radiation caries by increase in *Streptomutans, Lactobacillus, Candida* microorganism, and thick, acidic, viscous, small volume of saliva causes radiation caries.

Treatment of Xerostomia

- Use of sialogogues will stimulate the saliva secretion.
- Sugarless gum or candies stimulate secretion.
- Pilocarpine 15 mg/daily stimulates the secretion of saliva by acting on the salivary acinar cell receptors.
- Bromohexine can be used effectively in case of dry mouth due to SjÖgren's syndrome.
- A radioprotector such as amifostine can be used prior to the radiation to prevent the salivary dysfunction and reduce the severity of radiation oral mucositis.
- Mouth-wetting agents or saliva substitutes may be used when salivary stimulation is not possible, e.g. methylcellulose. It has excellent lubrication and inhibits the growth of microorganisms and maintained pleasant taste.

Teeth

During tooth developmental period: Retards the growth of teeth.

Before tooth calcification: Destroy the tooth bud.

After tooth calcification: Inhibits cellular differentiation, causing malformations and arresting tooth growth

- Children receiving radiation therapy to the Jaws show, defects in the permanent dentition such as retarded root development dwarfed teeth and anodontia.
- Teeth irradiated during development may complete calcification and erupt prematurely.
- Irradiation of teeth may retard root formation but no changes in the eruptive mechanism of teeth.
- Adult teeth are very resistant to the irradiation.
- Pulpal tissue shows fibroatrophy after radiation.
- Radiation causing no effect on enamel, dentin and cementum.

Radiation Caries

Radiation caries is a rampant form of dental caries that may occur in individuals who receive radiotherapy. Carious lesions result from changes in the salivary glands and saliva, including decrease in flow rate, pH level and buffering capacity. Increase in viscosity because of reduced or absent cleansing action of normal saliva results in accumulation of debris quickly. Radiation caries is the rapid course and widespread attack that distinguish other caries.

Clinically, three types of radiation caries exist:

1. The most common are widespread superficial lesions attacking, buccal, occlusal, incisal and palatal surfaces.
2. Involves the cementum and dentin in the cervical region **(Fig. 2.2)**.
3. Dark pigmentation of the entire crown.

Treatment plan for radiation caries is:

- Daily application of topical 1% sodium fluoride gel for 5 minutes in custom-made trays which causes delay in elevation of *Strepto-mutans* and *Lactobacillus.*
- Restoration of carious tooth.
- Maintains the good oral hygiene.
- Teeth with gross caries are often extracted before irradiation.
- Chlorhexidine rinses may reduce the level of *Streptococcus mutans* organisms.

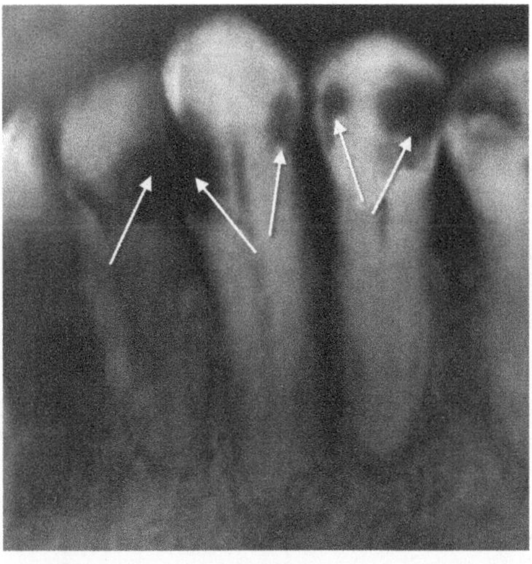

Fig. 2.2: Radiation caries involving cervical regions of teeth

Bone

Irradiation of the bone causes damage to the vasculature of the periosteum and cortical bone. Radiation also destroys osteoblasts and lesser extent of osteoclasts. Bone marrow is replaced with fatty marrow and fibrous connective tissue. Marrow tissue becomes hypovascular, hypoxic and hypocellular.

Osteoradionecrosis

Osteoradionecrosis is the most serious clinical complication that occurs in bone after irradiation. The decreased vascularity of the mandible renders, it easily infected by microorganisms from the oral cavity. This bone infection may result from radiation-induced breakdown of mucous membrane from denture sore or tooth extraction.

More common in mandible because of less vascular supply and more frequently exposed to irradiation Usually, large radiation doses are required for osteoradionecrosis to occur (e.g. <3000–5000 cGy) and changes may occur within a year after radiotherapy **(Fig. 2.3)**.

Treatment of osteoradionecrosis

- Prevent radiation caries by restoring all carious lesions before irradiation starts.
- Maintenance of good oral hygiene
- Daily topical fluoride application.

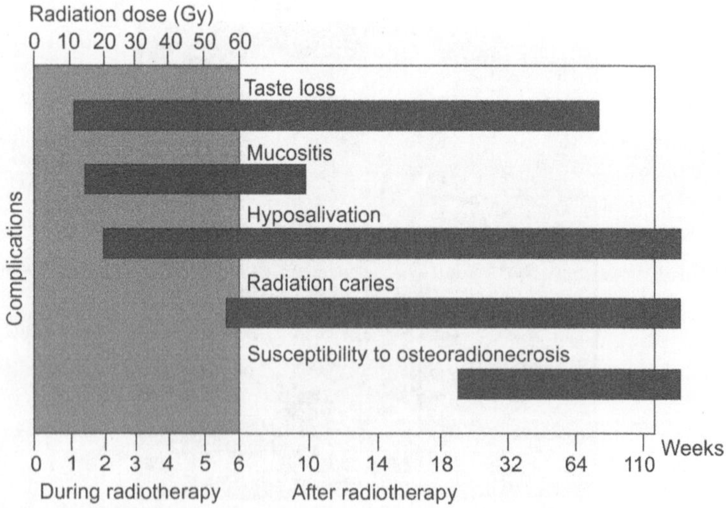

Fig. 2.3: Complications of radiotherapy with dosage and duration

- Remove all poorly supported and badly carious teeth and allow 7–14 days and up to 21 days sufficient time to heal ups the extraction wounds
- Adjusting dentures to minimize risk of denture sores.
- Hyperbaric oxygen (HBO) therapy may increase the oxygenation of tissues and angiogenesis, which promote osteoblastic and fibroblastic activity.
- Mucocutaneous flaps.
- Resection of sequestra or mandibulectomy.
- Nutrition supplements.
- Suitable antibiotics such as gentamycin or lincomycin and analgesics can be given.

BIOLOGIC EFFECTS OF WHOLE BODY IRRADIATION

When the whole body is exposed to low or moderate doses of radiation, characteristic changes develops (called acute radiation syndrome) **(Table 2.2)**.

Acute radiation syndrome: It is a collection of signs and symptoms experienced by the persons after whole body exposed to radiation **(Table 2.3)**.

Clinical manifestations depend on radiation dose:

Dose (Gy)	*Manifestation*
1–2 Gy	Prodromal symptoms
2–4 Gy	Mild hematopoietic symptoms
4–7 Gy	Severe hematopoietic symptoms
7–15 Gy	Gastrointestinal symptoms
50 + Gy	Cardiovascular and CNS symptoms

Prodromal symptoms: 1–2 Gy dose of radiation develops anorexia, nausea, vomiting, diarrhea, weakness and fatigue. Severity and time of onset depends on dose. Higher the dose, more rapid the onset and severity of symptoms.

Hematopoietic syndrome: Whole body exposure of 2–7 Gy cause injury to the hematopoietic stem cells of bone marrow and spleen causes, fall in the number of circulating granulocytes, platelets and finally erythrocytes.

The clinical signs are:

- Infection
- Hemorrhage (due to thrombocytopenia)
- Anemia (due to depletion of erythrocyte).

Table 2.2: Summary of the main acute effects following large whole-body doses of radiation

Dose	*Whole-body effect*
0.25 Sv	Nil
0.25–1.0 Sv	Slight blood changes, e.g. decrease in white blood cell count
1–2 Sv	Vomiting in three hours, fatigue, loss of appetite, blood changes. Recovery in a few weeks
2–6 Sv	Vomiting in two hours, severe blood changes, loss of hair within two weeks, recovery in one month to one year for 70%
6–10 Sv	Vomiting in one hour, intestinal damage, severe blood changes Death in two weeks for 80–100%
> 10 Sv	Brain damage, coma, death

Table 2.3: The effective X-ray dose of dental radiographic examinations

Radiographic examinations	*Effective dose (μSv)*
Full mouth periapical with D-speed, round collimator	150
Full mouth periapical with E-speed, rectangular collimator	33
Panoramic (Conventional)	4.0–10.0
Panoramic (Digital)	2.4–6.2
Cephalometric (Conventional)	2.3
Cephalometric (Digital)	1.6–1.7
Background radiation	3 mSv/yr or 8 μSv/day

When death results from the hematopoietic syndrome, usually occurs 10–30 days after irradiation.

Gastrointestinal syndrome: 7–15 Gy of whole body exposure causes loss of the epithelial layer of the intestinal mucosa, denuded mucosal surface leads to loss of plasma and electrolytes and reduce intestinal absorption occurs. All these changes are responsible for diarrhea, dehydration and loss of weight. Endogenous intestinal bacteria invade the denuded surface, producing septicemia.

Cardiovascular and CNS syndrome: Excess of 50 Gy exposures causes death in 1 to 2 days and other findings are collapse of the circulatory system:

- Decrease in BP
- Necrosis of cardiac muscle

Table 2.4: The estimates risk per million of developing a fatal radiation inducing malignancy from various X-ray examinations, based on present evidence

X-ray examination	*Risk per million of a fatal cancer*
Dental intraoral	0.2
Chest (male)	0.27
Chest (female)	0.47
Dental panoramic tomography	1.0
Skull	1.7
Lumbar spine	2.5
Pelvis	3.9
Abdomen	9.5
Barium meal	26
Barium enema	37
CT lung (male)	198
CT lung (female)	395

- Stupor, in coordination, disorientation and convulsions suggestive of extensive damage to CNS.

Radiation effects on embryos and fetuses: They are more radiosensitive than adults because embryonic cells are undifferentiated and high mitotic rate. Prenatal irradiation leads to death or specific developmental abnormality. Increase risk of childhood cancer such as leukemia and solid tumors.

Late somatic effects: Most important somatic effects are radiation-induced cancers **(Table 2.4)**. All radiation-induced cancers, other than leukemia show the following features:

- Most cancer appears approximately 10 years after exposure.
- Risk of exposure in childhood is more than the risk in adulthood.

Other late somatic effects:

- Impairment of growth and development results in reduced height, weight and skeletal development
- Mental retardation
- Induction of opacities in the lens of the eye.

PREVENTION AND MANAGEMENT OF RADIATION SIDE EFFECTS

There are several methods being utilized for the prevention of radiation therapy side effects. These mainly include altering the manner in which radiation is delivered and administering drugs that protect normal cells from radiation damage.

Radiation Delivery Methods

Two delivery methods that were originally used to reduce radiation side effects include dose fractionation, or splitting the total dose of radiation therapy into multiple doses and physical shielding with lead blocks to reduce the area of exposure.

- *Fractionation and hyperfractionation:* Radiation therapy was originally given in one large dose. More than a half-century ago, it was found that it was less toxic and more effective to administer radiation on a daily basis, a method called dose fractionation. Fractionation allows the delivery of a larger total dose of radiation to the cancer than would have been possible as a single dose. Currently, most radiation treatments are administered daily, 5 days a week. The 5 days per week is strictly for the convenience of maintaining a normal work week. The 24-hour interval and the two-day interval between doses allows for recovery of normal tissues between doses while cancer cells, in general, have less capability for recovery. There is no doubt that using fractionation has reduced side effects compared to single-dose delivery.

  While cancer cells tend to be less resilient than normal tissues, there is a chance that the intervals between fractionated doses of radiation may allow cancer cells to recover. Recent findings indicate that some cancers are best treated by reducing the 24-hour interval between doses to 6–8 hours, in order to enhance the toxic effects on cancer cells, while still preserving an adequate time interval for the recovery of normal cells. This technique, called hyper fractionation, is being widely used to treat a variety of cancers. Hyperfractionation requires sophisticated equipment, and therefore it is important for patients to be treated at specialty medical centers that have experience and staff trained in this technique.
- *Intensity modulated radiation therapy:* Intensity modulated radiation therapy (IMRT) delivers varying intensity of radiation with a rotating device. The intensity is varied by the placement of "leaves," which either block or allow the passage of radiation. The rotating component of this technique allows for more specific targeting of the cancer, sparing normal tissues from damage due to radiation exposure. In conventional radiation therapy, the beam is usually delivered from several different directions, possibly 5–10. The greater the number of beam directions, the more the dose will be confined

to the target cancer cells, sparing normal cells from exposure. IMRT delivers radiation from every point on a helix, or spiral, in contrast to only a few points.

IMRT is similar to CT scanning. In CT, a beam rotates around the patient, creating a sequence of cross-sectional images. IMRT also uses a rotating beam, except the beam delivers radiation. IMRT also delivers treatment one cross-section at a time.

- *Three-dimensional conformal radiation:* Three-dimensional conformal radiation therapy is a promising approach for the treatment of some cancers with decreased toxicity to normal tissues. Using computerized tomography (CT) scans and other scans, radiation oncologists have developed methods for determining the tumor size and shape in three dimensions. This allows high-dose external beam radiation therapy to be delivered primarily to the cancer with less damage to normal cells. It is important for conformal radiation to be administered at special cancer centers with sophisticated equipment and trained staff.

Drug Therapy

While preventing radiation side effects from occurring is the ideal approach to management, sometimes side effects are inevitable. In these situations, several types of drugs can be used to decrease the side effects of radiation. Drug therapies for radiation-induced side effects fall into two categories:

1. Those that protect the noncancerous tissue from radiation damage through systemic administration.
2. Those that are applied topically to mucus membranes to decrease or treat radiation damage.

Radioprotectors: Radioprotectants are drugs that selectively protect normal cells, but not cancer cells, from the effects of radiation **(Table 2.5)**.

- *Ethyol:* Ethyol is a radiation protector and the only drug that has been approved by the FDA for xerostomia (dry mouth) in patients receiving radiation therapy for cancers of the head and neck. Xerostomia is a chronic dry-mouth condition, which is caused by damage from radiation therapy to the salivary glands. Xerostomia can greatly impair a patient's ability to speak, chew, swallow and taste, and therefore, can have a negative effect on a patient's quality of life.
- *Steroids:* Steroids are naturally occurring hormones produced by the adrenal glands. Steroids such as prednisone or decadron (generic

Table 2.5: Radioprotectors and their mechanism of action

Category	*Radioprotectors*	*Mechanism of action*
Sulfhydryl compounds	Cysteine, cystamine glutathione, AET, WR 2127 and other WR-compounds.	Free-radical scavenging, donation of H atom.
Antioxidants	Tempace, Hoechst 33342,Vitamin A, E, and C, TMG and Melatonin	Free-radical scavenging
ACE inhibitors	Captopril, Elanopril, Pencillamine and Pentoxyfylline	Protease inhibition (through reninangiotensin system), anti-oxidation collagen synthesis inhibition
Cytoprotective agents	Mesna, dexrazoxane, amifostin (WR2127)	Reduced toxicity of chemotherapeutic drugs, decrease of urothelial toxicity and nephrotoxicity
Metalloelements	Manganese chloride, Cadmium salts, Bismuth Subnitrate, etc.	Metallothionine induction
Immunomodulators	Gamma-interferon, Polysaccharides AM5, AM218, Heat killed *Lactobacillus* cells, Broncho-Vaxom, Trehalose dicorynomycolate, AS101	Immune stimulation, increased production of cytokines
Lipopolysaccharides	Prostaglandins	Prostaglandin synthesis and elevated levels of cyclic AMP, DNA repair
Plant extracts and isolated compounds	Curcmin, Orientin, Vicinin	Free-radical scavenging, anti-oxidation
DNA-binding ligands	Hoechst 33342	Electron transfer, free-radical scavenging
Other compounds	Melatonin, Carnosin, Tempace, and Tempol	Free-radical scavenging Antioxidant, free radical scavenging

name is dexamethasone) drugs help decrease swelling in body tissues. Dexamethasone has also been shown to prevent radiation-induced vomiting, especially in treatment of cancers of the abdomen.

- *Topical agents:* Some drugs can be applied topically to mucus membranes to decrease or treat radiation damage. The topical agent sucralfate may protect mucus membranes by several mechanisms and is often used during and after radiation therapy for the prevention and treatment of mucositis (mouth sores). Topical antiseptics, such as chlorhexidine or benzydamine, have been used for the prevention of mucositis, but recent research indicates that these are not effective. Chlorhexidine was found to be more toxic, and no more effective than placebo in the prevention of mucositis. German researchers reported that chlorhexidine mouthwashes were not effective in treating mucositis in patients with a low white blood cell count. Despite a significant decrease in the aerobic and anaerobic bacterial flora on the oral mucous membranes, the risk of mucositis seemed to be enhanced. The patients treated with chlorhexidine seemed to have more problems with inflammation, resulting in mucositis.

Strategies to Improve Prevention and Management of Radiation Side Effects

Future progress in the prevention and management of radiation side effects will result from the continued evaluation of new treatments in clinical trials. Areas of active investigation aimed at improving the prevention and management of radiation side effects include the following:

- Keratinocyte growth factor (KGF, palifermin)
- Antioxidants
- Interleukin 11
- Prostaglandins

Keratinocyte Growth Factor (KGF, Palifermin)

This is a growth factor that has been shown to stimulate growth of epithelial cells, which make up the mucus membrane and line the mouth and throat. Keratinocyte growth factor is currently being tested in patients to prevent chemotherapy damage to the mucus membranes of the gastrointestinal tract.

Antioxidants

The antioxidant agent Cu/Zn superoxide dismutase (SOD) has shown promise in reducing early and late radiation-induced tissue injury.

Interleukin 11

Interleukin 11 is a growth factor that is similar but not identical to what the body normally produces. Interleukin 11 has been approved by the FDA to stimulate platelet recovery in patients with low platelet counts due to chemotherapy.

Prostaglandins

Prostaglandins are a group of compounds that affect the healing of inflammation and wounds. Misoprostol is a prostaglandin that is effective in treating complications that arise in patients with prostate cancer who receive radiation treatment.

CHAPTER

3

Radiation Safety and Protection

Many potential risks associated with the use of ionizing radiation such as (a) stochastic, and (b) nonstochastic effects.

Stochastic effects: Probable chance of radiation effect occurs, e.g. *leukemia.*

Nonstochastic effects: Definitive radiation effects occur, e.g. skin rashes, cataract and infertility.

To prevent these radiation effects, there are some radiation protection measures to use radiation safely. The aim of radiation protection is to minimize the radiation exposure to the patient as well as office personnel. Philosophy of radiation protection is based on the rules. *ALARA—As low as reasonably achievable.*

Radiation protection can be divided into:

- *Radiation protection to the patient*
- *Radiation protection to the operator*
- *Radiation protection to the other public.*

RADIATION PROTECTION TO THE PATIENT

It can be divided into:

- Patient selection
- Choice of equipment
- Choice of intraoral technique
- X-ray equipment
- Processing the film
- Interpretation of the image.

Patient Selection

Professional judgment should be used to select the patient for X-ray examination; such criteria could reduce the number of unproductive radiographic examinations and thus protect the patient from unnecessary radiation.

Choice of Equipment

Choice of equipment includes:

- Selection of the image receptor (X-ray film)
- Focal spot to film distance
- Collimation
- Filtration
- Use of leaded aprons and collars.

Image Receptor Selection

- Faster films (E-speed) are routinely used to reduce the exposure time **(Fig. 3.1)** without sacrifice of image quality (Speed of the film depends on the size of the silver halide crystals. Larger crystals have greater speed and vice versa).
- Use of double-sided emulsion to reduce the exposure.
- Use double film packets to reduce 50% radiation reduction compared to single film packets.
- Xeroradiographs can be used to produce good image quality with reduced radiation exposure.
- Intensifying screens are used in extraoral radiography could dramatically reduced exposure time **(Fig. 3.2)**.
- Green emitting (rare earth elements such as Gadolinium and Lanthanum) intensifying screens are 8 times more sensitive to X-rays than blue emitting (calcium tungstate) intensifying screens thus required a less radiation exposure.

Focal Spot-film Distance

In intraoral radiography, two techniques are used bisecting angle and paralleling cone technique. In bisecting, focal spot to film distance is 8 inch but 16 inch in case of paralleling cone technique. Skin exposure

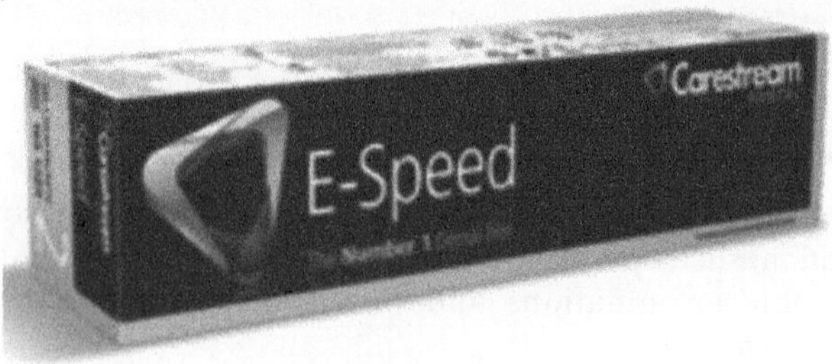

Fig. 3.1: E-speed X-ray film
Courtesy: Kodak.co

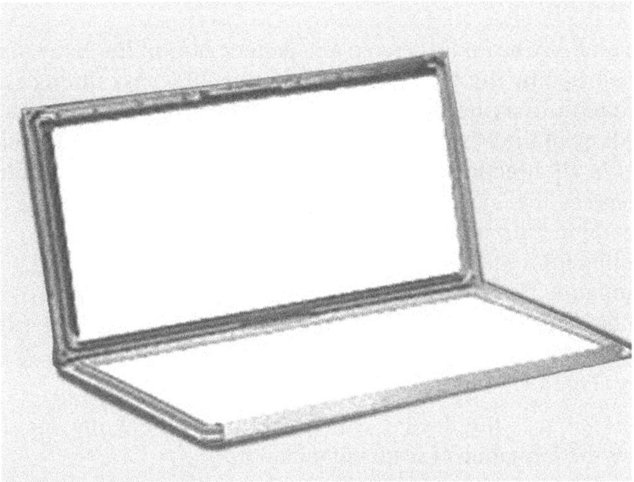

Fig. 3.2: Intensifying screen with cassette for panoramic radiography

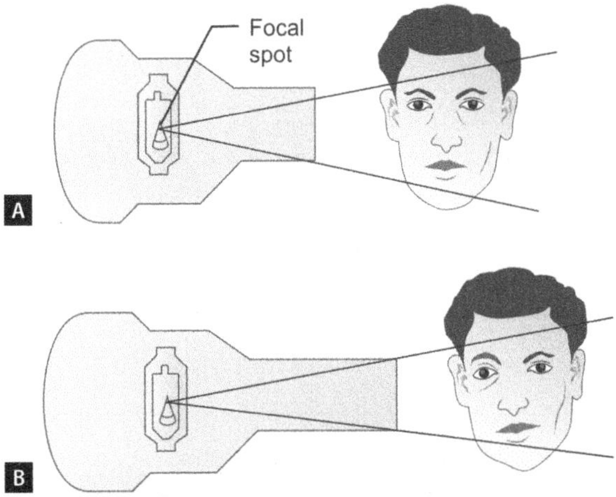

Figs 3.3A and B: Effect of focal spot to object distance. (A) In bisecting (short cone) technique larger area of skin irradiated; (B) Small area irradiated in paralleling (long cone) technique

is decreased with the long focal spot to film distance; this is because at the long distance the X-ray beam is less divergent and small focal spot size thus reducing the area of exposure. But in case of bisecting angle technique, distance between target to film is 8 inch results in more diverging X-rays causing more skin area get exposed **(Figs 3.3A and B)**.

Collimation

When an X-ray beam is directed at a patient, 90% of the X-ray photons are absorbed by the tissues and remaining 10% pass through as the information carrying beam results in the formation of image on a film. Many of the absorbed photons generate scattered radiation that travels in all directions because of Compton effect results in film fog and degrade the image contrast. To reduce this problem placing a lead collimator in the path of the X-ray beam.

Collimation means reduces the size of the X-ray beam by placing a radiopaque *(lead)* barrier containing aperture in the path of beam and thus reduces the volume of irradiated tissue by absorbing scattered radiation there by reduces patient exposure and increases the film quality **(Figs 3.4A and B)**.

Collimator: It is the device, which collimates the X-ray beam thus reduces the formation of scattered radiation.

Three types of collimators are used **(Figs 3.5A to C)**:

1. Diaphragm
2. Tubular
3. Rectangular

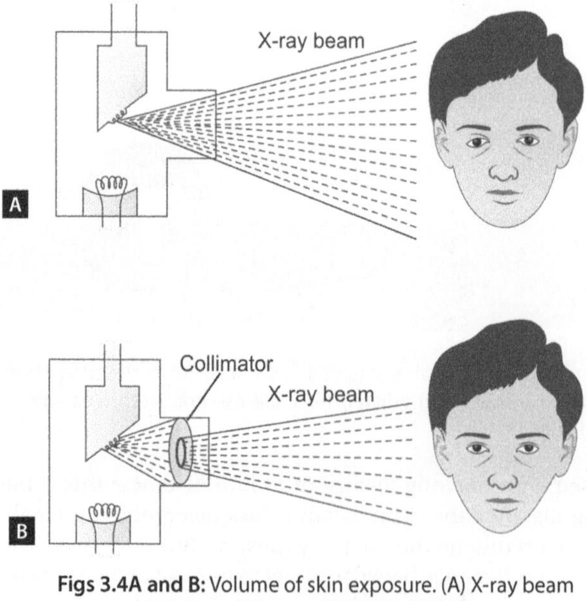

Figs 3.4A and B: Volume of skin exposure. (A) X-ray beam without collimator; (B) with collimator

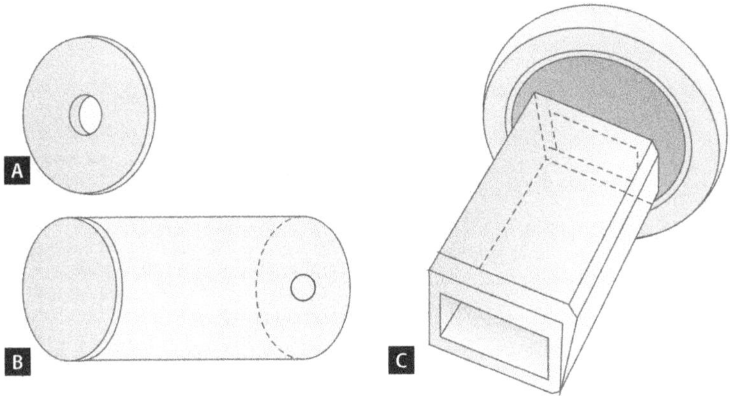

Figs 3.5A to C: Types of collimator. (A) Diaphragm collimator; (B) Tubular collimator; (C) Rectangular collimator

By using collimators, only 7 cm of the patient skin surface can be irradiated thus prevent the unwanted area of the body.

Filtration

X-ray beam emitted from the X-ray tube consists of not only high energy (short wavelength) but also low energy (long wavelength) photons. Low energy photons have little penetrating power and they are absorbed within the tissues causing hazard to the patient and gives no contribution to the image formation over the film. The purpose of adopting filtration is to selectively remove these low energy photons from the X-ray beam by placing an aluminum filter in the path of the beam and allows high energy photons which results in reduced patient exposure.

Two types of filtration:
1. Inherent filtration
2. External filtration

a. *Inherent filtration:* This filters the X-ray beam within the X-ray machine by glass wall of the X-ray tube, insulating oil that surrounds the X-ray tube and barrier material that prevents the oil escaping out. The inherent filtration of X-ray machine is equivalent to 0.5–2 mm of aluminum. Inherent filtration alone does not meet the standard regulated by federal law, therefore external or added filtration is required.

b. *External filtration:* Total filtration is the sum of the inherent filtration plus added external filtration applied in the form of *aluminum* discs placed in the path of X-ray beam **(Figs 3.6A and B)**.

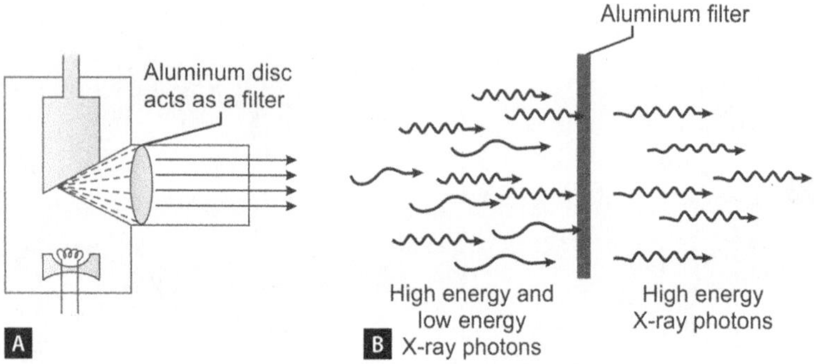

Figs 3.6A and B: (A) Aluminum disc in the path of X-ray beam; (B) Filters stops the low energy photons and allows the high energy photons

Further patient exposures may be reduced by removing both low and high-energy X-ray photons, allowing mid-range energy photons to expose the film. This can be achieved by using rare earth elements such as *Samarium*. The use of this material result in almost 40% reduction in patient exposure as compared with conventional aluminum filters.

Leaded Aprons and Collars

Leaded aprons, collars and gloves should be used to minimize any unnecessary radiation exposure **(Figs 3.7A to C)**. Philosophy of radiation protection is based on the principle of *ALARA (As Low As Reasonably Achievable)*. According to this principle even the small dose would cause some deleterious effects to reduce this use a leaded aprons and thyroid collar which absorbs 94% of the scatter radiation.

Choice of Intraoral Techniques

Paralleling cone technique has a less skin exposure than the bisecting angle technique because in parallel cone technique focal spot to film distance is more therefore, X-ray beams are projecting more parallel to each other. But choice of technique depends on the diagnostic quality of the resultant radiographs and more efficient the technique reduces the retakes of radiographs thereby reduce the patient exposure.

X-ray Equipment

X-ray generating equipment includes the selection of appropriate machine, kVp, mA and exposure time.

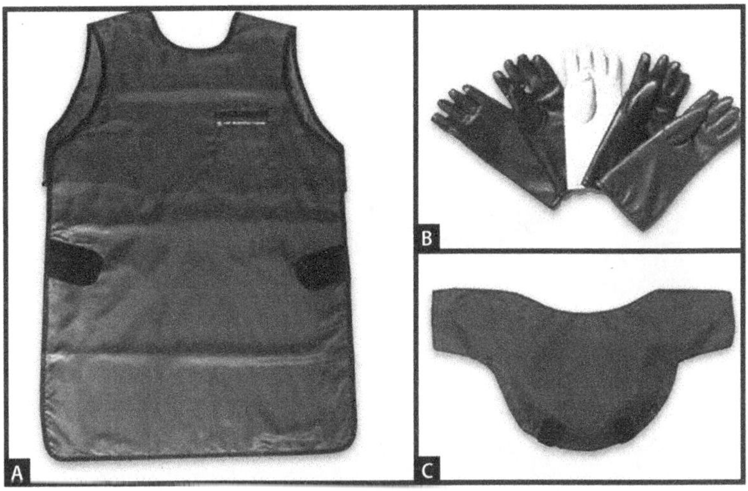

Figs 3.7A to C: (A) Lead apron; (B) Lead gloves; (C) Thyroid collar

Kilovoltage: It is the voltage potential difference between the anode and the cathode of X-ray tube. The higher the kVp the greater the potential difference, more will be the attraction of electrons by the anode and greater will be the energy (quality) of the photons, thus the kVp will produce X-ray photons with more penetrating power.

When kVp increased there will be greater energy in the photons and the less such photons are required to expose the film, which reduces the exposure time to maintain the film density. kVp also affects the radiographic contrast. Increase the kVp produces more scattered radiation and thus further reducing the contrast of the image but greater the contrast in case of lower the kVp.

Milliampere: It is the amount of current, which is passed through the X-ray tube. It is directly proportional to the number of production of X-ray photons. mA will lead to increased in the number (quantity) of photons.

Exposure time: Exposure time will produce more X-ray radiation that causes hazards to the patient. In practice to reduce the exposure times and maintains proper kVp and mA without loss of contrast of the radiographs. Exposure time mainly affects the:

- Density
- Contrast of a radiograph

Density is the overall degree of darkening of the exposed film. Increase the exposure time will lead to more darkening (density) of the film and vice versa.

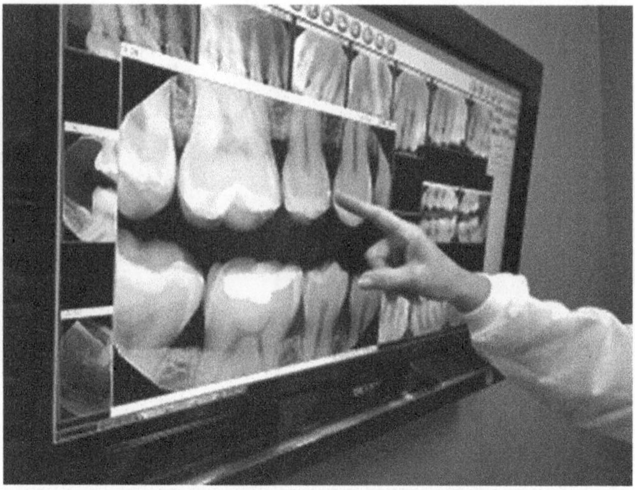

Fig. 3.8: Interpretation of radiographic image

Contrast is the difference in density between various regions on the film. Increase exposure time results in high contrast and vice versa.

Processing the Film

Major cause of unnecessary repeat the radiograph due to improper processing like, over developing (dark radiograph) and under developing (light radiograph) which results in inferior diagnostic quality of the image. Use of proper method in processing significantly reduces the retake, which prevent the patient from radiation exposure.

Interpretation of Image

Radiographic images should be viewed under proper conditions to obtain maximum available information. Radiographs should be viewed in a semidarkened room with light transmitted only through the films **(Fig. 3.8)**. This type of radiographic study prevents the remaking the film. Thus protect the patient from radiation exposure.

RADIATION PROTECTION TO THE OPERATOR

- Every effort should be made so that the operator can leave the room or take a position behind a suitable barrier or wall during exposure of the film and wall must be sufficient density or thickness (minimum thickness should be 9 inch wall) so that exposure would be prevented.

- Operator should stand at least 6 feet away from the X-ray source at an angle of 90–135° to the central ray of the X-ray beam to protect from the radiation because according to inverse square law, intensity of the beam diminishing as the distance (minimum 6 feet) increased and scatter radiation will be absorbed by the patient head at an angle of 90–135° **(Fig. 3.9)**.
- Films should never be held intraorally by the operator. Ideally film-holding instruments should be used such as artery forceps, snap-a-ray, bite blocks and XCP film holders **(Figs 3.10A to D)**.
- The operator or patient should not stabilize X-ray tube during the exposure.
- Operator should use personnel monitoring devices such as film badge or thermoluminescent dosimeter to measure the occupational exposure **(Figs 3.11A and B)**.

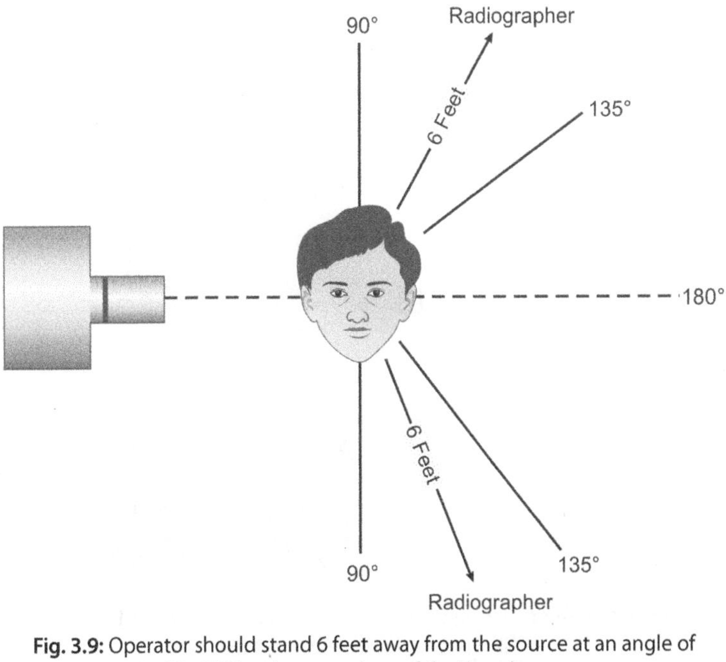

Fig. 3.9: Operator should stand 6 feet away from the source at an angle of 90–135° to the central ray of the X-ray beam

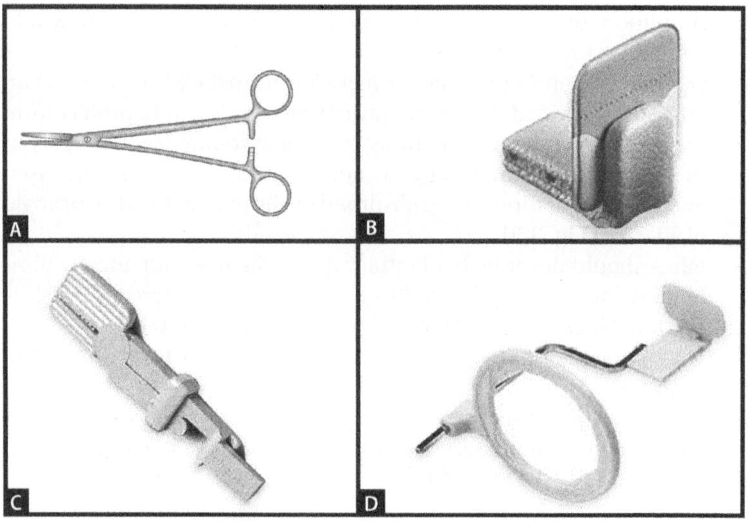

Figs 3.10A to D: Intraoral film holding instruments. (A) Artery forceps; (B) Bite blocks; (C) Snap-A-ray; (D) XCP film holder

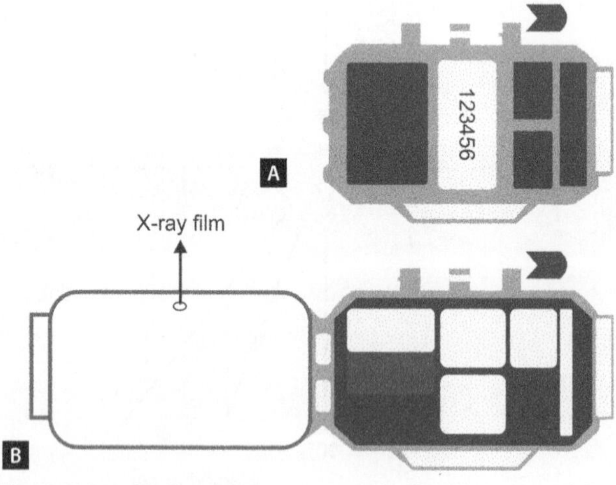

Figs 3.11A and B: Personnel monitoring device. (A) Unopened device; (B) Opened device with X-ray film

RADIATION PROTECTION TO THE PUBLIC

- X-ray room wall should line with lead or walls constructed of gypsum or painted with barium have been found to be adequate for the average dental office.
- Other than patients should not enter the radiology room.
- Warning sign boards have to be displayed outside the radiology room.

CHAPTER 4

Quality Assurance in Dental Radiography

Quality assurance is a plan of action to ensure that a diagnostic X-ray facility will produce consistent, high-quality images with a minimum of exposure to patients and personnel.

Quality assurance means regular testing to detect equipment malfunctions, planned monitoring and scheduled maintenance for consistent film processing, and regular assessment of other variables that affect image quality.

The benefits derived from a quality assurance program far outweigh implementation efforts and costs. In addition to aiding in diagnosis, a well carried out quality assurance program results in minimized radiation dosage to patients because radiographs are produced under the most favorable conditions.

QUALITY CONTROL TESTS

Quality control tests are specific tests that are used to maintain and monitor dental X-ray equipment, supplies, and film processing. To avoid excess exposure of patients and personnel to X-radiation, the dental radiographer must have a clear understanding of the quality control procedures used to test specific equipment, supplies, and film processing in the dental office.

Equipment and Supplies

Quality control tests are necessary to monitor:

- X-ray equipment and accessories
  - Dental X-ray machine,
  - Dental X-ray film,
  - Screens and cassettes, and
  - Viewing equipment.
- *Film processing:* To consistently produce diagnostic quality radiographs, dental X-ray equipment and supplies must be functioning properly and kept in good working condition.

DENTAL X-RAY MACHINES

All dental X-ray machines must be inspected and monitored periodically. Some state and local regulatory agencies provide dental X-ray equipment inspection services as part of their registration and licensing procedures. Dental X-ray machines must also be calibrated, or adjusted for accuracy, at regular intervals. Calibration of dental X-ray equipment must be performed by a qualified technician to ensure consistent X-ray machine performance and the production of diagnostic radiographs.

Quality control tests for dental X-ray machine should be performed annually. These tests are designed to identify minor malfunctions, including machine output variations, inadequate collimation; tube-head drift, timing errors, and inaccurate kilovoltage and milli-amperage readings (AERB has well-laid norms, which are a mandate to follow in every radiology facility).

In addition to regular calibration, the American Academy of Oral and Maxillofacial Radiology recommends that the following eight tests of X-ray generating equipment be conducted annually:

1. X-ray output
2. Kilovoltage (kVp) calibration
3. Half-value layer
4. Timer
5. Milliamperage (mA)
6. Collimation
7. Beam alignment
8. Tube head stability.

Checking the Quantity of X-ray Beam (X-ray Output Test)

The purpose of checking the quantity of the X-ray beam is to verify that, the output of the X-ray machine has not changed since the last exposure. The quantity of X-ray photons is affected by mA circuit and by the exposure time. The measure for quantity of X-ray beam, the X-ray machine is set at a standardized set of exposure parameter, i.e. 0.25 sec (15 impulses), 7 or 10 mA, and 65 or 70 kVp, and measure the quantity of radiation generated using radiation dosimeter.

Checking the Timer

The purpose of checking the timer is to see whether it is functioning accurately. This procedure can also be used to demonstrate the principle that X-rays are generated in impulses in self-rectified dental X-ray machines.

Checking the mA Circuit

The purpose of checking the mA circuit is to ensure the proper functioning of the 10 and 15 mA settings on dental X-ray machines. If the dental X-ray machine has only one mA setting (usually 7 mA) the mA circuit can be checked using an ammeter.

Checking the Penetrating Power of X-ray Beam (Half-value Layer Test)

The purpose of checking the penetrating power of X-ray beam is to ensure that the kVp circuit is functioning within safe limits. This procedure can be used to visibly demonstrate the half-value layer (HVL) principle that states: "50% of the X-ray photons should penetrate through a standardized thickness of a given material (usually aluminum) depending on kVp." The quality or penetrating power of the X-ray beam is measured by its half-value layer. The standard that is set by the federal government states that if the X-ray machine has a maximum of 69 or less kVp, 50% of the X-ray output must pass through at least 1.5 mm thickness of aluminum; if the X-ray machine delivers 70 or more kVp, then 50% of the X-ray output must pass through at least 2.5 mm of aluminum.

Checking the Accuracy of the kVp Setting

The purpose of checking the kVp is to determine the accuracy of kVp settings on the dental X-ray machine. A kVp meter is used to check the kVp.

The machine is set at any kVp setting or the maximum kVp setting and aimed at the target area on the kVp meter. The exposure time should be long enough for the kVp meter to obtain a reading (1 second or 60 impulses). The kVp meter measures the wavelength and frequency of the beam of radiation and gives an accurate kVp, regardless of the setting of the machine. The measured kVp should be the same as X-ray machine setting. If it is different, the problem is associated with the X-ray machine, not the external power supply to the dental office.

Checking the Focal Spot

The purpose of checking the focal spot is to evaluate the surface area of the focal spot that becomes pitted over time and enlarges. An enlarged focal spot decreases sharpness and increases magnification. Focal spot size can be checked by using a test object containing a number of bar patterns to test the resolution of the image. A small focal spot provides sharpness that is measured by resolution. When X-ray machine is new, the focal spot is relatively small, and the eye can resolve about 11–12 line pairs per millimeter. However, as the focal spot degrades, the resolution decreases to seven or less line pairs per millimeter, and the image gets fuzzy or unsharp.

Checking the Collimation of the X-ray Beam

The purpose of checking the collimator is to ensure proper collimation of the beam. According to Federal standards, the beam of radiation must be collimated to 2.75 inches at the tip of position-indicating device (PID).

Collimation test: To test collimation, place the PID of X-ray machine against a rare earth fluorescent screen or a loaded panoramic cassette. The exposure time is set at about 1 or 2 seconds. The lights in the room are then turned off; observe through the leaded barrier window to see if the fluorescence is limited to the diameter of the PID; or process the panoramic film to check, if the exposed area of the film is limited to the diameter of the PID. Collimation can also be verified by placing four size 2 dental X-ray film in the form of a cross-shaped template **(Figs 4.1A and B)**. Expose the films using bite-wing settings, process the films, and reconstitute the pattern. The size and alignment of beam then can be determined.

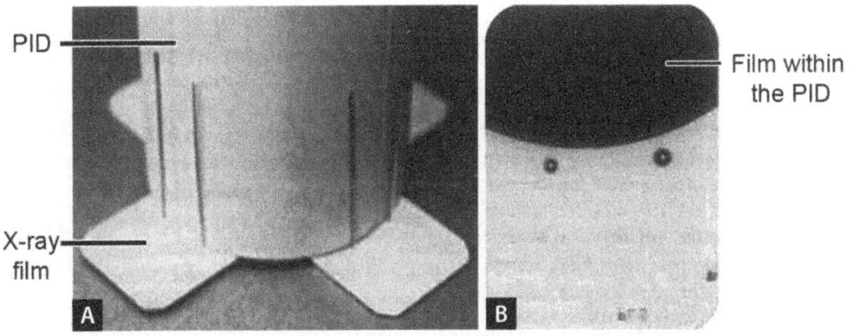

Figs 4.1A and B: (A) The alignment of the collimation of the X-ray beam and end of the aiming cylinder can be checked by making a cross-pattern of film, centering the aiming cylinder, making the periphery with needles, and making an exposure; (B) One of the processed radiographs showing the dark exposed area just inside the holes. If this pattern is seen on all films, then good alignment is demonstrated

Checking the Tube Head Stability

The tube head should be stable, when place around the patient's head and not drift during an exposure. When it is not stable, service is necessary to adjust the suspension mechanism.

DENTAL X-RAY FILM

Dental X-ray film is quite stable when properly handled. The dental X-ray film must be properly stored in a cool, dry facility and away from a radiation source. Use the dental X-ray film before its expiry date.

Fresh film test: Unwrap one unexposed film from a newly opened box and process using fresh processing solutions. If the processed film appears clear with a slight blue tint, the film is fresh and has been properly stored and protected. A film that has expired, has been improperly stored, or has been exposed to radiation appears fogged and it must not be used.

SCREENS AND CASSETTES

The intensifying screens used within extraoral film cassette should be examined periodically for the presence of scratches and dirt. Monthly cleaning of intensifying screens is important with commercially available cleaners as recommended by the screen manufacturer. Screens that appear visibly scratched should be replaced. Cassette holders must be examined for worn closures, light leaks, and warping, which may result in fogged and blurred radiographs; such cassettes must be replaced or repaired. Cassettes must also be checked for adequate screen-film contact.

Screen-film contact test: Insert one film between the screens in the cassette holder. Place a wire mesh test object on top of the loaded cassette. Position the PID using a 40-inch target-film distances while directing the central ray perpendicular to the cassette. Expose the film using 10 mA, 70 kVp, and 15 impulses. Process the exposed film. View the film on a view-box in a dimly lit room at a distance of 6 feet. If the wire mesh image seen on the film exhibits a uniform density, it reveals adequate screen-film contact. If the wire mesh image seen on the film exhibits varying densities, it reveals inadequate screen-film contact. Areas of poor screen-film contact appear darker than good contact areas.

VIEWING EQUIPMENT

The view-box, or illuminator, is a light source that is used to view dental radiographs. The view-box contains fluorescent light bulbs that emit light through an opaque plastic or plexiglass front. The view-box should emit a uniform and subdued light for proper radiographic interpretation. The photographic light meter can be used to determine proper viewing brightness. The view-box should be periodically examined for dirt and discoloration of the plexiglass surface. The surface of the view-box should be cleaned weekly. Permanently discolored plexiglass surface must be replaced. Any burnt fluorescent light bulbs must also be replaced.

FILM PROCESSING

Film processing is one of the most critical areas in quality control because deficiencies in this process are the most potential cause of nondiagnostic radiographs. Quality control tests must be performed routinely to determine the acceptable conditions for film processing; which greatly increases the likelihood of producing radiographs of consistently high quality.

Darkroom Lighting

The darkroom must be inspected monthly to assess the light leaks and integrity of safelights. Film may become fogged in the darkroom from inappropriate safelight filters, excessive exposure to safelights, and stray light from other sources. Such films are dark, show low contrast, and have muddy gray appearance. The following " light-leak test" and "coin test" or "penny test" can be recommended monthly to evaluate for fogging caused by light-leak and inappropriate safelight conditions.

Light-leak test: Close the darkroom door and turn off all lights, including the safelights. Once the eyes are accustomed to the darkness, observe the areas around the door, walls and ceiling, the vent areas, and the keyhole for light leaks. If present, mark the light leaks with chalk or masking tape. Light leaks must be corrected with weather stripping or black tape before proceeding with film processing.

Penny test or coin test: Unwrap an exposed film and place the test film on the area where films are usually unwrapped and clipped on the film hanger (at least 4 feet from the safelight).

Place the coin on the film and allow the film and the coin in this position for usually 5 minutes, approximate time required to unwrap and mount a full-mouth set of films in dark room. Remove the coin and process the test film as usual. If the image of the coin and a fogged background appears on the resultant film, the room is not light safe **(Figs 4.2A and B)**. Light-leak and safelight problems should be corrected before proceeding with film processing.

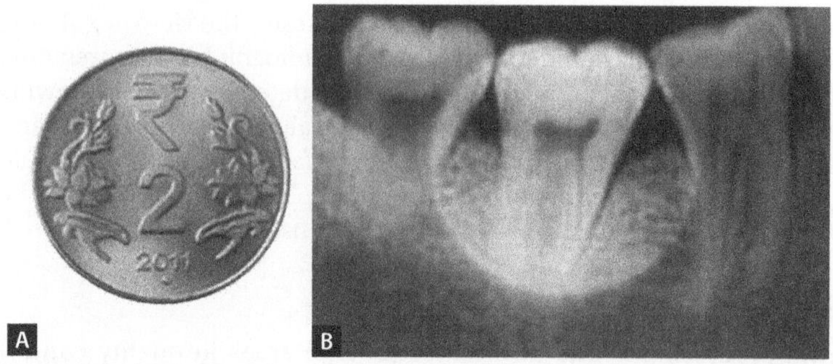

Figs 4.2A and B: Coin test/Penny test for unsafe illumination. (A) Unwrap and place a coin on the exposed film on the working surface for about 5 minutes in dark room; (B) If the processed radiograph shows an outline of the coin, the film is being fogged by inappropriate safelight conditions

Processing Equipment

Manual and automatic processing equipment must be meticulously maintained and monitored on the weekly basis, because deficiencies in the processing are the most common cause of faulty radiographs. The thermometer and timer must be checked for accuracy, level of water in the bath, developer and fixer solutions must also be monitored in manual processing techniques. The time-temperature recommendations for the processing must be strictly followed.

If automatic processing equipment is used, the water circulation system, the solution levels, replenishment system, and temperatures must be monitored. The manufacturer's procedure and maintenance directions must be carefully followed.

Automatic processor test: Unwrap two unexposed films and expose one to light. Process both the films in automatic processor. If the unexposed film appears clear and dry and the film exposed to light appears black and dry, the automatic processor is functioning properly. If the automatic processor is not functioning properly, then the processing solutions and dryer temperature must be checked.

Processing Solutions

The most critical component of film processing quality control is the monitoring of processing solutions. The processing solutions must be replenished daily; the developer should be replenished with fresh developer or with developer replenisher and the fixer should be replenished with fixer. The processing solutions should be replaced depending primarily on the rate of use of the solutions; usually every second week. The processing solutions must be evaluated each day before any patient radiographs are processed.

DEVELOPER STRENGTH

When the developer solution loses its strength, the time-temperature recommendations of the manufacturer are no longer accurate. The strength of the developer can be checked by comparing film densities to a standard. The following tests can be used:

- Reference radiograph
- Step-wedge radiograph
- Normalizing device.

Reference Radiograph

A reference radiograph is a simple and effective means for constant monitoring of the quality of images. A reference radiograph is one that is, exposed using ideal exposure factors, processed under ideal conditions, with optimal density and contrast, and then used to compare film densities of the radiographs that are processed everyday. All the subsequent radiographs are compared one beside another with this reference film mounted on the view-box. If the regular radiographs appear light and have reduced contrast than the reference radiograph, the developer solution is either weak or cold. If the regular radiographs appear darker than the reference radiograph, the developer solution is either too concentrated or too warm. Weakened or concentrated solution must be replaced, and if the developer solution is too cool or too warm, the temperature must be adjusted.

Step-wedge Radiograph

Step-wedge radiograph provides an accurate monitoring of day-to-day processing conditions. It measures the speed of the imaging system and image contrast. A step-wedge is a device constructed of layered aluminum steps. When a step-wedge is placed on the film and exposed to X-rays, the different steps absorbs varying amounts of X-rays. When processed, different film densities can be seen on the radiograph as a result of the step-wedge. A step-wedge can also be readily made by using the lead foil from the film packets. Stack five sheets together and staple at one end; cut-off 4/5 of the top layer, 3/5 of second layer, 2/5 of third layer, and 1/5 of fourth layer. This creates a four-step wedge. Place the wedge

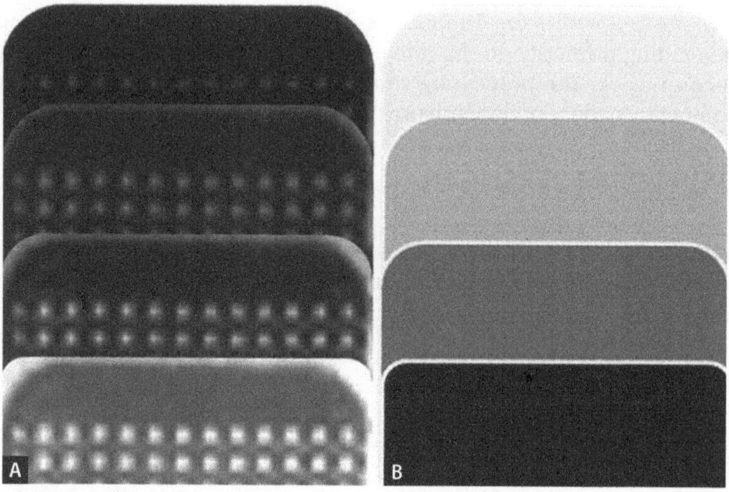

Figs 4.3A and B: (A) Step wedge made of strips of lead foil from film packets. This step wedge is positioned over a film, and an exposure is made; (B) Processed radiograph showing each step. Such an image should be made daily after replenishing processing solutions and compared with an image made with fresh solutions. When the step wedge has become one full step lighter, it is time to change the processing solution

on top of a film and expose; the resultant radiograph show four steps from dark to light **(Figs 4.3A and B)**. Compare the densities seen on the daily radiograph with densities on the standard step-wedge radiograph on the view-box. When the density on the daily radiograph differs from that on the standard radiograph, then the developer solution is depleted and should be changed before proceeding with processing.

Normalizing Device

Normalizing and monitoring device can be used to monitor developer strength and film density.

FIXER STRENGTH

The fixer solution removes the unexposed silver halide crystals and results in "clear" areas on the processed dental radiograph. When the fixer solution loses its strength, the film takes a longer time to clear. The strength of fixer can be monitored by clearing test.

Clearing Test

Unwrap a film and place it immediately in the fixer solution. Check the film for clearing and clock the amount of time taken. If the film is not completely clear after 2 minutes, re-immerse it in the fixer solution. If the film does not completely clear in 3 to 4 minutes, the fixer solution is depleted. The fixer solution should be replaced before proceeding with processing **(Table 4.1)**.

Summary of several quality assurance tasks should be performed daily, weekly, monthly and yearly to ensure ideal radiographs as given in **Table 4.2**.

Table 4.1: Quality control tests for film processing

Day	*Solution strength*	*Quality control tests*	*Test results*
1	Use fresh, full-strength processing solutions	*Reference radiograph:* Using correct exposure factors expose and process one film. This film becomes the "reference radiograph." *Step-wedge radiograph:* Expose 21 step-wedge films; process one film. This film becomes the "standard radiograph"	The reference radiograph demonstrates optimal film contrast and density The standard radiograph demonstrates optimal film contrast and density
2, 3, etc.	Fresh processing solutions weaken with time and use; exhausted solutions result	*Reference radiograph:* Each day, expose and process one film to compare with the reference radiograph *Step-wedge radiograph:* Each day, process one of the previously exposed step-wedge films.	Compare the daily film with the reference radiograph: • If densities match, continue processing. • If densities do not match, replace processing solutions. • Compare the daily film with the standard radiograph: • If densities match, continue processing. • If densities differ by one full step on the step wedge, replace processing solutions.

Table 4.2: Schedule of quality assurance procedures

Daily • Compare radiographs with reference film • Enter findings in retake log • Replenish processing solutions • Check temperature of processing solutions • Make step-wedge test of processing system
Weekly • Replace processing solutions • Clean processing equipment • Clean view boxes • Review retake log
Monthly • Check darkroom safe lighting • Check intensifying screens • Rotate film stock • Check exposure charts
Yearly • Calibrate X-ray machine

CHAPTER 5

X-ray Films and Techniques

X-ray film or image receptor is a type of photographic film and is of two types

1. Intraoral X-ray film (Direct exposure film).
2. Extraoral X-ray film or screen film (Indirect exposure film). (discussed detail in extraoral radiography chapter)

Intraoral X-ray Film

This type of film is sensitive primarily to X-ray photons.

Composition: X-ray film composed of two principal components **(Fig. 5.1)**.

1. Emulsion
2. Base

Emulsion: It is sensitive to X-rays and visible light and records the image. Emulsion contains 2 ingredients.

1. Silver halide crystals
2. Gelatin matrix.

Silver halide crystals composed of mainly silver bromide and lesser content of silver iodide which are photosensitive and increase the photosensitive further by adding sulfur contaminant and each silver grains diameter is 0.7–0.75 mm.

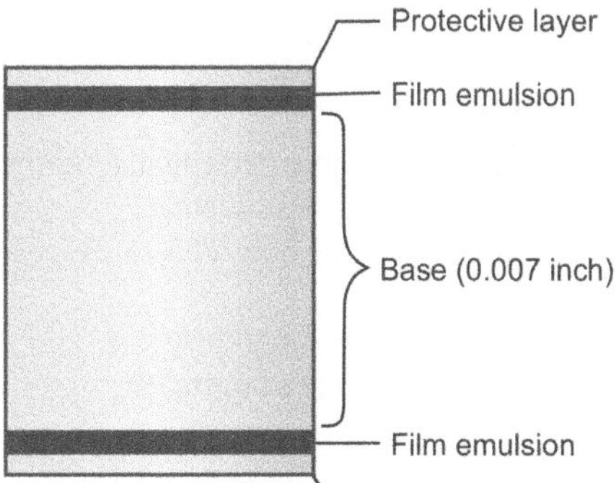

Fig. 5.1: Cross section of X-ray film

Gelatin matrix suspends silver halide crystals evenly in the gel made from cattle bone. Gelatin absorbs the processing solution thus allowing the chemicals to react with the silver halide crystals.

Protective coat overlying the emulsion is an additional gelatin layer protects the film from damage by scratching, contamination and pressure from the rollers during automatic processing.

Base: It is made up of polyethylene terephthalate (polyester) with 0.2 mm (0.007 inch) thickness. The function of the base is to support the light sensitive silver halide crystals. Base is slightly blue tint to enhance the image quality.

Film speed: Speed refers to the amount of radiation required for the crystals to produce a radiographic image of standard density.

Speed is controlled by the size of the silver halide crystals. Larger size of silver halide crystals required less radiation there by increases the film speeds and vice versa. The speed of X-ray film is indicated by a letter A B C D E F. The fastest dental film currently used are, Kodak ultra speed film (Group D) and Kodak Ekta speed film (Group E). Ekta speed film requires half the exposure of ultra-speed film.

Image Sharpness

Image sharpness depends mainly on size of the silver crystals, the smaller the crystals size finer the image sharpness. Slow speed films have small size crystals and faster films have larger crystals size.

INTRAORAL RADIOGRAPHY

Intraoral radiographs are of three categories on basis of their clinical applications:

1. Periapical radiography
2. Bitewing radiography
3. Occlusal radiography.

Periapical Radiography

In periapical radiographic technique, periapical films are used to record the crown, root and periapical regions of teeth.

Five different sizes of intraoral X-ray films **(Fig. 5.2)** are available among them,

- Size # 0-2 used for periapical radiography
- Size # 3 exclusively for bitewing radiography
- Size # 4 for occlusal radiography.

1. Size # 0 → for small children (pedo film) 22 × 35 mm.
2. Size # 1 → for adult anterior projections 24 × 40 mm.

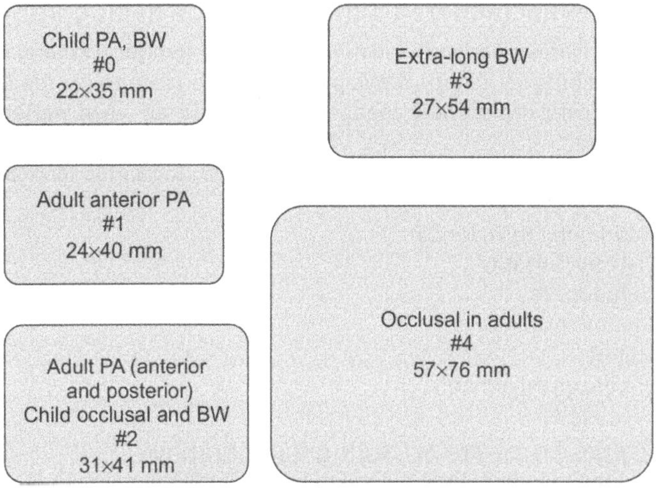

Fig. 5.2: Different intraoral film sizes
Abbreviations: PA, periapical; BW, bitewing

3. Size # 2 → standard films for adults 31 × 41 mm.
4. Size # 3 → standard bitewing films for adults 27 × 54 mm
5. Size #4 → occlusal films in adults 57 × 76 mm.

Indications for Periapical Radiographs

- To evaluate the dental caries.
- To evaluate the periapical infections.
- To evaluate the periodontal diseases.
- To evaluate the mixed dentition analysis.
- Assessment of root morphology before extraction.
- To evaluate the small neoplasm and cysts especially in periapical region.
- To evaluate the pathology of bone in periapical area.
- To evaluate the pulpal calcification and pulp stones.
- To evaluate the dental anomalies.
- Assessment of working length in endo treatment.
- To evaluate the impacted teeth.

Limitations

- In patient with difficulty in opening the mouth (trismus).
- Patient with gagging sensation while taking posterior region of teeth.
- Larger cyst and tumor that cannot be covered completely by periapical film.

Difficulties Encountered during Periapical Radiography

Lot of difficulties is encountered during intraoral periapical radiography. Similar technique is not always possible often need to be modified in periapical radiographic technique to obtain an ideal periapical radiographs.

Problems encountered during periapical radiographic techniques are:

- Mandibular third molars
- Gagging sensation
- Endodontics
- Edentulous patients
- Children
- Handicapped patients.

Difficulties Encountered during Radiography of Mandibular Third Molars

The main problem is placement of the X-ray film sufficiently posteriorly into the lingual sulcus so that film has to cover the apical edges of impacted third molar (particularly when it is horizontally impacted) and avoid the gagging reflex.

Possible solutions:

- Ask the patient to relax deeply before taking radiographs.
- Clip top of the X-ray film to film holder (snap-A-ray holder for bisecting angle technique or extension care paralleling (XCP) holder for paralleling technique) in such a way that only half of the film holder is use to hold the X-ray film instead of using full length of holder so that X-ray film can be sufficiently placed posteriorly to cover the distal part of impacted third molar without gagging reflex **(Fig. 5.3)**.
- To avoid gagging reflex, ask the patient to view some photographs or charts or ask them to concentrate on breathing deeply.
- In case of horizontal type of impaction, apex may not be recorded on the film by using ideal techniques (**Figs 5.4A and B**), in such cases modification has to be done to record the apex of the tooth. X-ray film is placed in the same position as before but the X-ray tube head is positioned further posteriorly (change in horizontal angulations without changing vertical angulations) aiming anteriorly to project the apex of the third molar on to the film **(Fig. 5.4C)**.

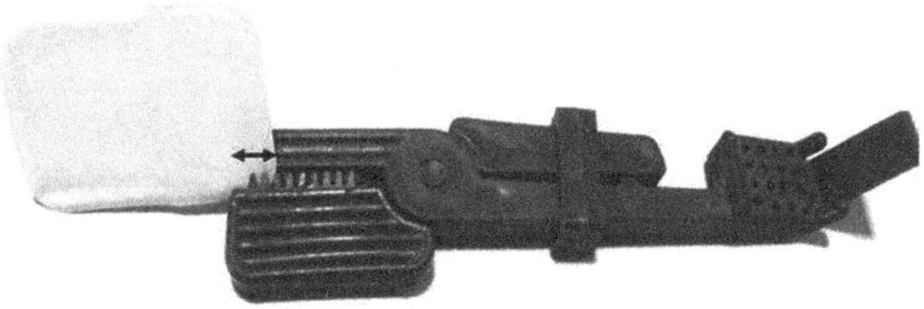

Fig. 5.3: X-ray film should be clipped to half of the snap-A-ray film holder so that film can be placed sufficiently posteriorly to cover the entire impacted teeth

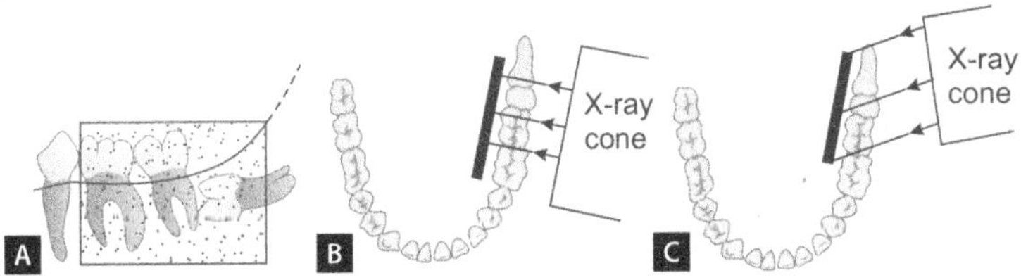

Figs 5.4A to C: Modified X-ray cone position for impacted third molar. (A) Radiograph showing part of impacted molar; (B) With normal cone projection; (C) Modified X-ray cone project anteriorly to cover the entire area of impacted molar

Problems of Gagging Reflex

The gag reflex is strong in some patients which prevents the placement of the film in the desired position particularly in posterior regions of both the jaws.

Solutions

- Spray the palate or lingual sulcus with local anesthetic before placing the X-ray film into the oral cavity.
- Ask the patient to view some photographs or charts or listening light music to divert patient mind.
- Ask the patient to concentrate on breathing deeply while taking radiographs.

Problems Encountered during Endodontics

The main difficulties are:

- Film placement and stabilization when endodontics instruments rubber dam, and clamps are in position.
- Identification and separation of root canals.
- Assessing root canal length in foreshortened or elongated radiographs.

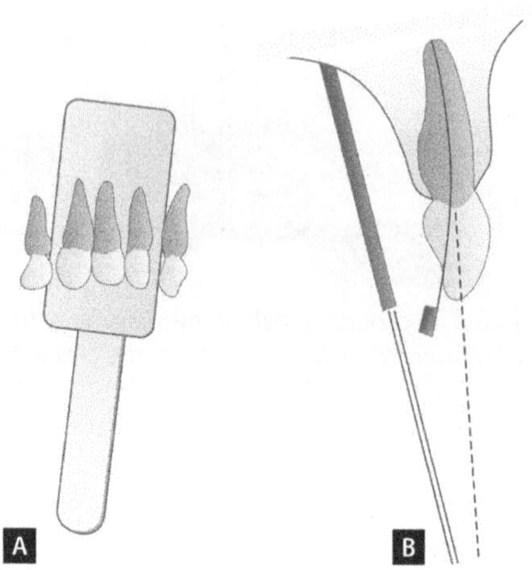

Figs 5.5A and B: Wooden spatula. (A) Front view showing X-ray film attached to the spatula and placed in desired area; (B) Side view of wooden spatula

Possible solutions: The problem with placement of the X-ray film and stabilization can be solved by X-ray film can be attached to wooden tongue spatula. This is positioned in the mouth in a desired place and held in place by the patient without disturbing the endodontic instruments as shown in **Figures 5.5A and B**.

The problem of identifying and separating the root canals can be solved by taking at least two radiographs using different horizontal angulations to avoid overlapping of the root canal as shown in **Figures 5.6A to D**.

The problem of assessing root canal length in fore-shortened or elongated image is very difficult to know the actual working length of the instrument. The possible solutions are:

- Using paralleling technique take a preoperative periapical radiographs and measures the length of the root directly from the radiograph. The amount of distortion on subsequent films using bisecting angle technique can be assessed.
- Calculating mathematically by actual length of a root canal from a distorted tooth image taken with a diagnostic instrument using bisecting angle technique by measuring the **(Fig. 5.7)**
  - Radiographic tooth length.
  - Radiographic instrument length.
  - Actual instrument length.

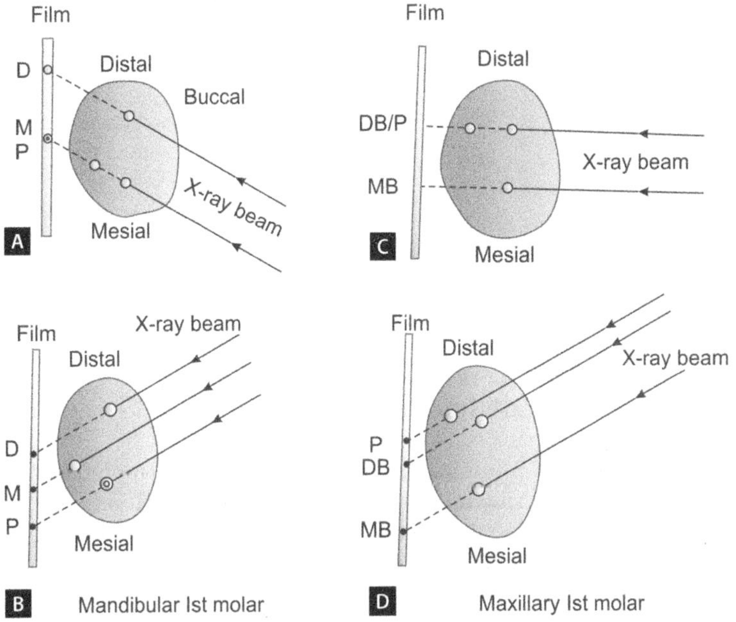

Figs 5.6A to D: Effect of different horizontal angulations to avoid overlapping of root canals. (A) Radiograph of mandibular 1st molar shows mesial and palatal canal are overlapped with usual horizontal angulation; (B) Different horizontal angulation appears separation of root canals; (C) Radiograph of maxillary 1st molar shows distobuccal and palatal root canals are overlapped; (D) Slight change in the horizontal angulation gives separation of root canals

Substitute the measurements into the formula

$$\text{Actual tooth length} = \frac{\text{Radiographic tooth length} \times \text{Actual instrument length}}{\text{Radiographic instrument length}}$$

Calculate the actual tooth length and adjust the working length of the instrument as necessary.

Problems in Edentulous Patient

The main problem in the edentulous or partially edentulous is placement of the X-ray film into the mouth.

In edentulous alveolar ridge, the depth of the lingual sulcus is reduced hence paralleling technique are not advisable. In such cases modified bisecting angle technique is performed. Assess the angle between the long axis of the alveolar bone and the X-ray film and X-ray tube position

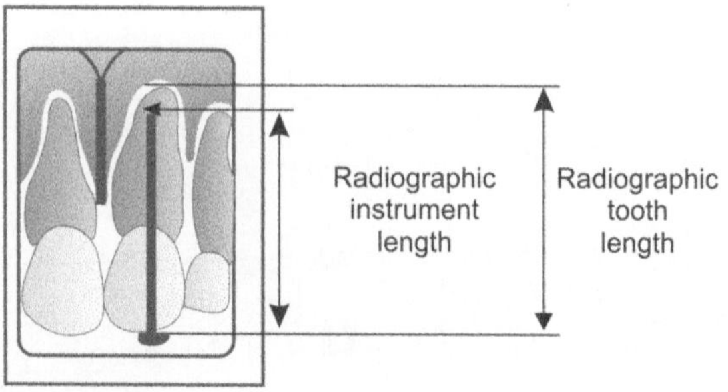

Fig. 5.7: Measurement of actual tooth length required in endodontics

adjusted accordingly so that X-ray beam must direct perpendicular to the bisector line which bisects the angle formed between the long axis of the bone and the film.

In partially edentulous patient, difficulties lie in the proper placement of the film holder without displacement. In such cases cotton rolls are to be placed in the edentulous area to support the film holder held in position **(Figs 5.8A and B)**.

Problems Encountered in Children

In children the problem is to place the X-ray film with holder into the mouth without movement.

The paralleling technique is not possible in small children but can often be used anteriorly for investigating traumatize tooth.

A modified bisecting angle technique is possible in most children, with the X-ray film placed flat in the mouth (occlusal plane) and the X-ray tube position is adjusted accordingly so that, X-ray beam directs perpendicular to the bisector line **(Fig. 5.9)**.

Problems with Handicapped Child

The problem encountered during radiography of handicapped child is, patient un-cooperation and possible anatomical difficulties in relation to film placement.

Possible solutions:

- Avoid taking unnecessary radiographs.
- If radiographs required, then using paralleling technique because with this technique the position of the film, teeth and X-ray beam are maintained irrespective of the patients head position.

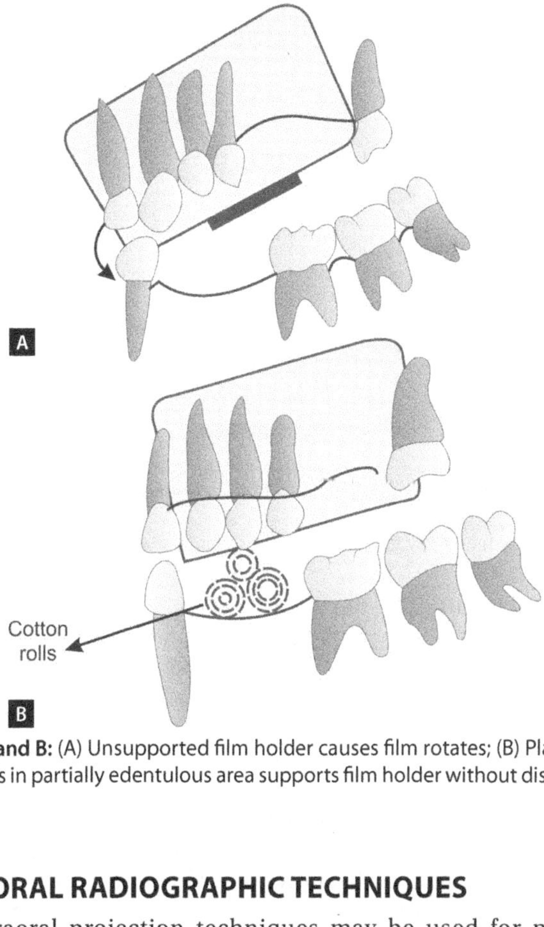

Figs 5.8A and B: (A) Unsupported film holder causes film rotates; (B) Placement of cotton rolls in partially edentulous area supports film holder without displacement

INTRAORAL RADIOGRAPHIC TECHNIQUES

Two intraoral projection techniques may be used for periapical radiography:

1. Bisecting angle or short cone technique
2. Paralleling cone or long cone technique or McCormack's or Fitzgerald or right-angle techniques.

Bisecting Angle or Short Cone Technique

The bisecting angle technique is based on a simple geometric theorem. Cieszynski's rule states that, two triangles are equal when they share one complete side and have two equal angles.

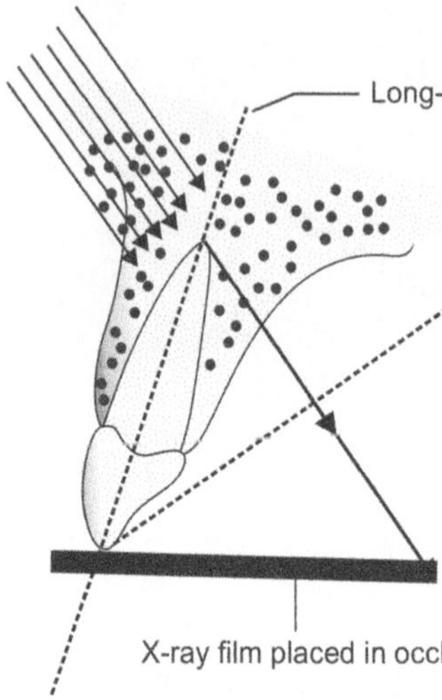

Fig. 5.9: Position of X-ray film in the occlusal plane and direction of X-ray beam

In dental radiography the theorem is applied as follows, the X-ray film is positioned as close as possible to the lingual or palatal surface of the tooth. The plane of the film and the long axis of the tooth form an angle, with its apex at the point where the film is in contact with the tooth. When this angle is bisected by an imaginary line two equal angles with a common side (imaginary bisector) is formed **(Fig. 5.10)**.

X-ray beam projected perpendicular to the bisector, which bisects the angle equally formed by the long axis of the tooth and the film. The formation of image will show distortion because the film and object are not parallel and the X-ray beam is not directed perpendicular to long axis of tooth and the film.

When the X-ray cone is directed at increased vertical angulation, the image appeared as foreshortened. If X-ray cone is directed at reduced vertical angulation results in elongation of the image. The target-to-object distance in this technique is 8 inch.

Vertical angulation for bisecting angle projections:

Projections:	*Maxilla:*	*Mandible:*
Incisor	+40°	–15°
Canine	+45°	–20°
Premolar	+30°	–10°
Molar	+20°	-5°

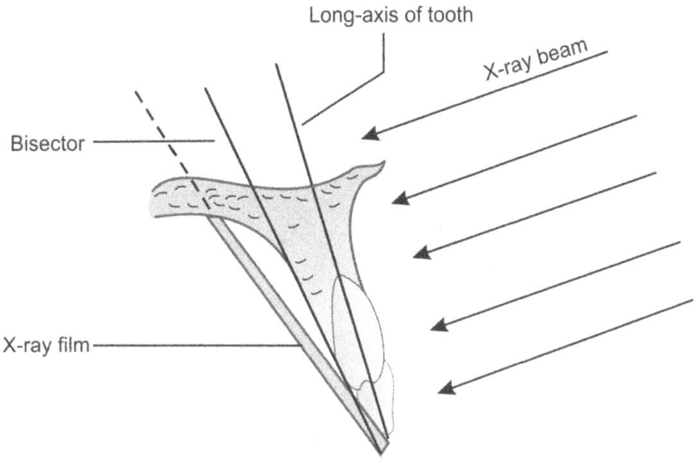

Fig. 5.10: In bisecting angle technique X-ray beam project at right angles to the imaginary bisector, which bisects the angle formed between long-axis of film and the tooth

Horizontal angulation: X-ray cone should be adjusted for proper horizontal angulations in such a way that, central ray should pass through the interproximal contact area of required tooth thus avoid the overlapping of adjacent tooth. The shape of the arch and the position of the teeth determine the horizontal angulation **(Fig. 5.11)**.

Patient head position: In maxillary radiographs, head should be little downward so that ala-tragus line parallel to the floor. In mandibular radiographic projections chin should be tilted upward so that line drawn from the corner of the mouth to the tragus of the ear should be parallel to the floor **(Figs 5.12A and B)**.

X-ray cone position: Horizontal and vertical planes are the two guide planes has to be considered for positioning the X-ray cone.

Maxillary Projection (Fig. 5.13A)

Horizontal plane: Line drawn from the ala of the nose to tragus of the ear.

Vertical plane: Vertical planes are drawn according to the interesting tooth.

- *Incisors:* vertical planes are drawn along the tip of the nose
- *Canine:* Ala of the nose
- *Premolar:* Mid pupillary line

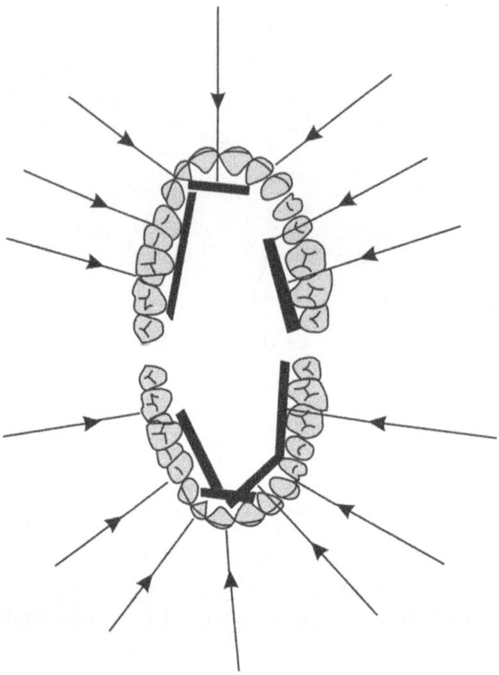

Fig. 5.11: Different horizontal angulation depends on the shape of the arch

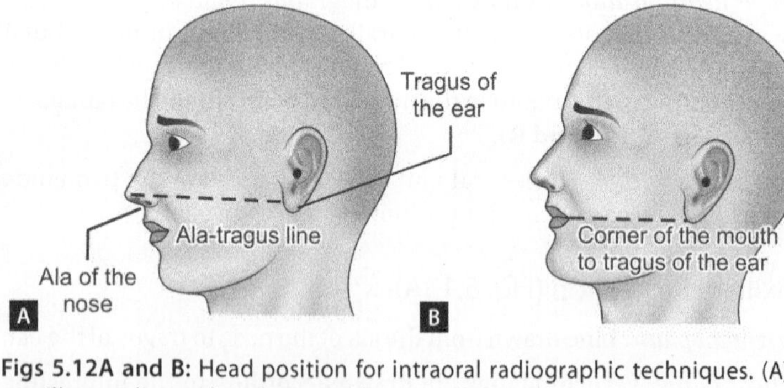

Figs 5.12A and B: Head position for intraoral radiographic techniques. (A) In maxillary radiography, ala-tragus line parallel to the floor; (B) In mandibular radiographic technique, line joining between the corner of the mouth to tragus of the ear

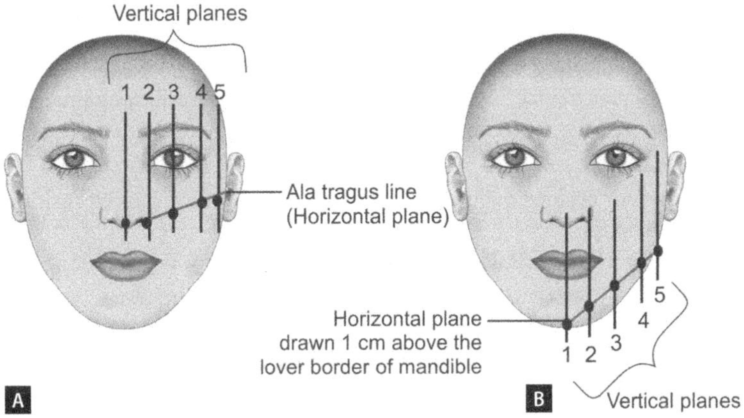

Figs 5.13A and B: (A) Maxillary radiography; ala-tragus (horizontal plane) line and the vertical plane drawn with respect to the each tooth, 1: vertical plane drawn along the tip of the nose, 2: ala of the nose, 3: mid-papillary, 4: outer canthus of the eye, 5: 1 cm away from the outer canthus of the eye. Black point indicates, X-ray beam insertion at particular each tooth, where horizontal and vertical planes are meet each other; (B) Mandibular radiography; horizontal plane drawn 1 cm above the lower border of mandible and the vertical planes are similar of maxillary radiography

- *Molar:* Outer canthus of the eye
- *Third molar:* 1cm away from the outer canthus of the eye.

X-ray cone should be positioned in a point where both the vertical and horizontal planes meet each other for a respected tooth.

Mandibular Projection (Fig. 5.13B)

Horizontal plane: Line drawn 1 cm above the lower border of the mandible.

Vertical plane: Vertical planes are drawn according to the interesting tooth, similar to the maxillary radiography.

- *Incisors:* vertical planes are drawn along the tip of the nose
- *Canine:* Ala of the nose
- *Premolar:* Mid-pupillary line
- *Molar:* Outer canthus of the eye
- *Third molar:* 1 cm away from the outer canthus of the eye.

Center of the X-ray cone should be positioned in a point where both the vertical and horizontal planes meet each other for a respected tooth.

Advantages:

- It is very comfortable for the patient.
- Film positioning is relatively simple and quick.
- No special device is necessary to positioning the film against the teeth.

Disadvantages:

- Improper vertical angulation results in foreshortening or elongation of the image.
- Improper horizontal angulation results in overlapping of teeth.
- Not possible to assess accurate dimension of the object.

Paralleling Cone Technique or Long Cone Technique

In this technique film is placed parallel to the long axis of the tooth **(Fig. 5.14)**. To achieve this parallel orientation of film and tooth, it is often necessary to position the film in middle of the oral cavity, i.e. away from the tooth by a special XCP film holder device. In this technique use a relatively long open-ended aiming cylinder (cone) to increase the focal spot to object distance, i.e. 12–16 inches. This permits more parallel rays of the beam to the film there by reducing the image magnification and increase the image sharpness and resolution.

Advantages of Paralleling Cone Technique

- Accurate image are produced with less magnification.
- For endodontic purpose to measure the accurate root canal length.

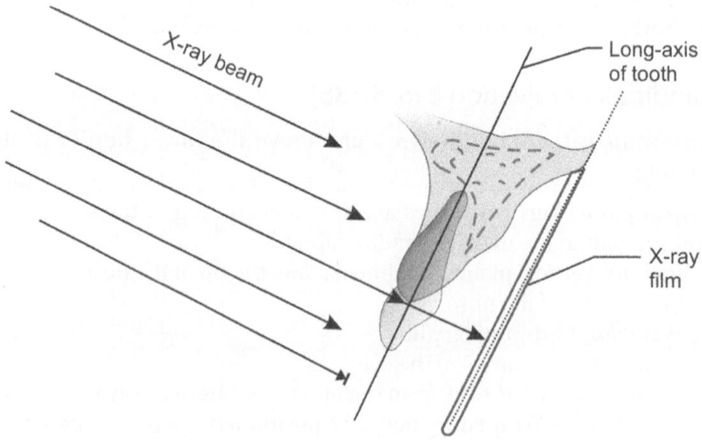

Fig. 5.14: In paralleling cone technique X-ray beam project exactly at right angles to the long-axis of the film and the tooth

Disadvantages

- Uncomfortable while placing the film holder in to the mouth.
- Unskilled technicians cannot be performed.

OBJECT LOCALIZATION OR CLARK'S TECHNIQUE

To determine the location of a foreign object or an impacted tooth with in the Jaws by *tube shift cone technique or Clark's rule or buccal object role or SLOB technique.*

Two radiographs of an object exposed. First radiograph taken at a usual horizontal angulation, i.e. called reference radiograph. Then second radiograph taken with slightly shifts the cone either mesial or distal to the usual angulation. If the object image moves in the direction of tube shifting indicates object lies in the lingual or palatal side and opposite movement of object shows that object in the buccal or labial aspect **(Figs 5.15A and B)**.

SLOB means: **S**ame side **L**ingual, **O**pposite side **B**uccal.

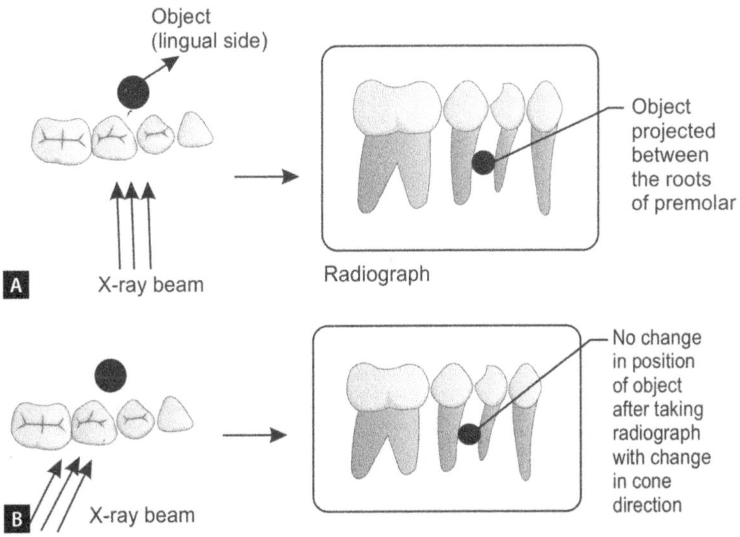

Figs 5.15A and B: SLOB technique revealed the location of foreign object. (A) Reference radiograph has taken with usual angulation shows object appeared between the roots of premolar; (B) X-ray tube shifted distally and checks for the position of object, the resultant radiograph shows no change in position of object indicates object lies on lingual side, if object moved opposite to the tube shifted indicates object lies on buccal side

BITEWING RADIOGRAPHY

In this radiographic technique periapical films are used to record the coronal portions of the maxillary and mandibular teeth in one image **(Fig. 5.16)**. In adult, size 2 or size 3 (27 × 54 mm) periapical films and size 1 for children's are usually used to take bitewing projection.

Bitewing films have a paper tab projecting from the middle of the film on which the patient has to bites to support the film **(Fig. 5.17)**.

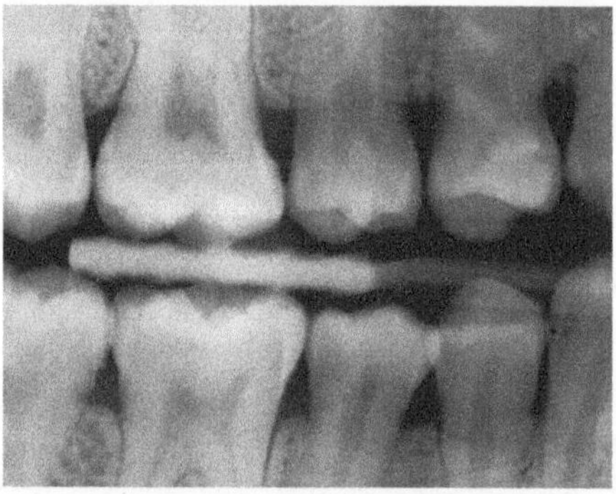

Fig. 5.16: Bitewing radiograph

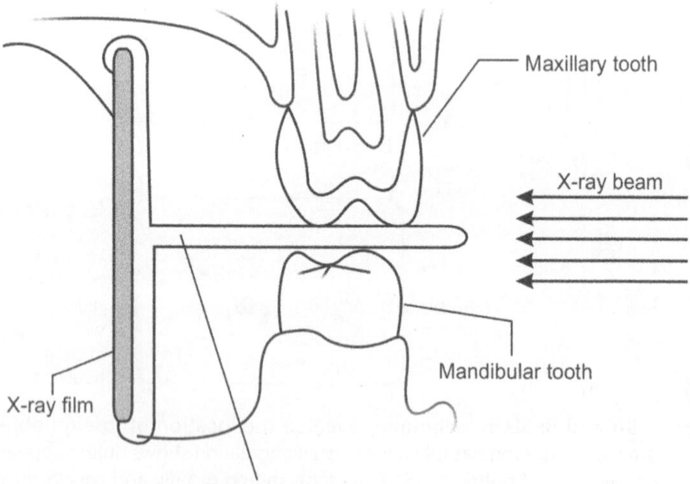

Fig. 5.17: Position of X-ray film and film holder with respect to upper and lower tooth in bitewing radiographic technique

Indications for Bitewing Radiography

- Mainly used to detect interproximal caries.
- To evaluate height of the alveolar crest in assessment of periodontal disease.
- Monitoring the progression of dental caries.

OCCLUSAL RADIOGRAPHY

Occlusal films are used to take larger areas of maxilla and mandible. Intra orally films are held in position by the patient bite lightly on the film to support it between the occlusal surfaces of each jaw.

Size of the film is 57 × 76 mm.

Indications of Occlusal Radiography

- To evaluate the impacted canine, third molar, and locate retained root stump and supernumerary tooth.
- To localize foreign bodies in the Jaws such as Sialolith in the ducts of salivary glands **(Fig. 5.18)**.
- To evaluate the integrity of the anterior border of the maxillary sinus.

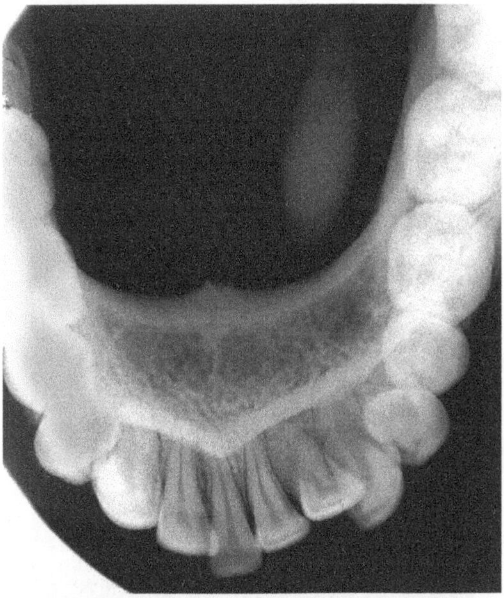

Fig. 5.18: Mandibular occlusal radiograph shows large sialolith in the submandibular duct

- Most useful in assessment of the periapical region in patient with trismus
- To detect complete extension of large cysts and tumors this cannot be covered completely by periapical radiographs.
- Assessment of fracture of the anterior teeth and alveolar bone.

There are three types of occlusal projections:
1. Topographical view of maxillary or mandibular jaws
2. Cross sectional view of maxillary or mandibular jaws
3. Lateral topographical occlusal projections.

Topographical (Anterior) View of Occlusal Projections

Primary field of this projection is anterior portion of jaws, i.e. from canine to canine. The central rays are directed towards the center of the film. The vertical angulation in maxillary is +45° and –55° for mandibular **(Figs 5.19 and 5.20)**.

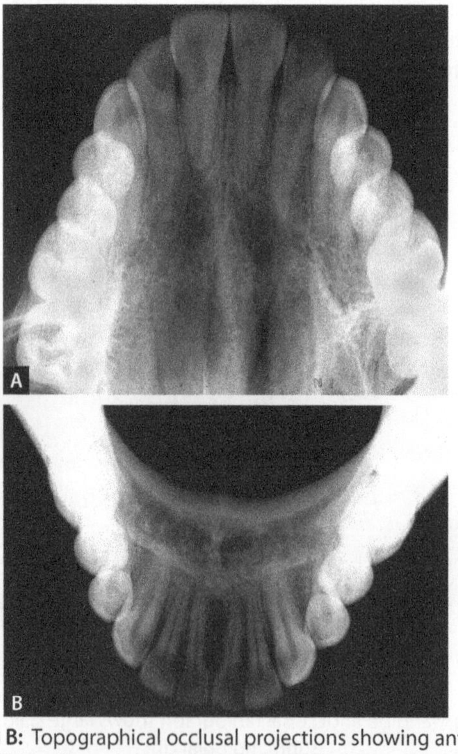

Figs 5.19A and B: Topographical occlusal projections showing anterior portions of teeth. (A) Maxillary occlusal view; (B) Mandibular occlusal projection

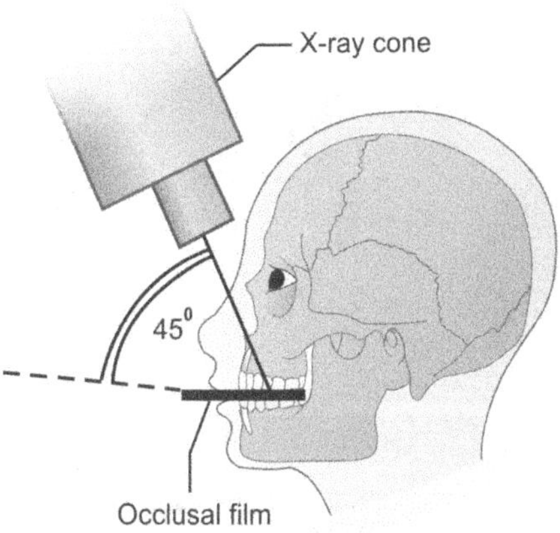

Fig. 5.20: Position of film and the X-ray cone in maxillary topographical occlusal projections

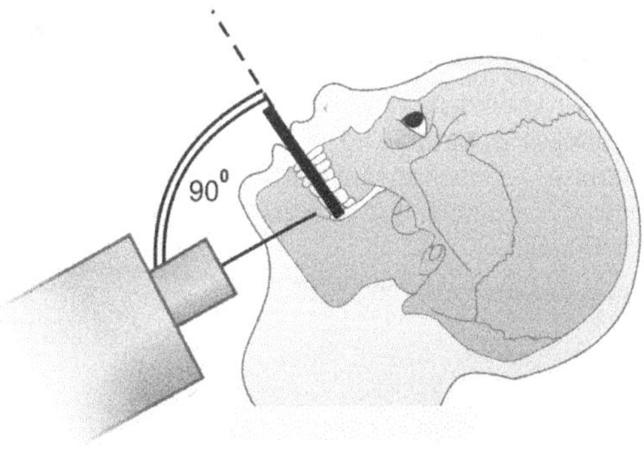

Fig. 5.21: True occlusal view of mandible

Cross-sectional (Posterior) View of Occlusal Projection

This projects the posterior aspects of jaws **(Figs 5.21 and 5.22)**.

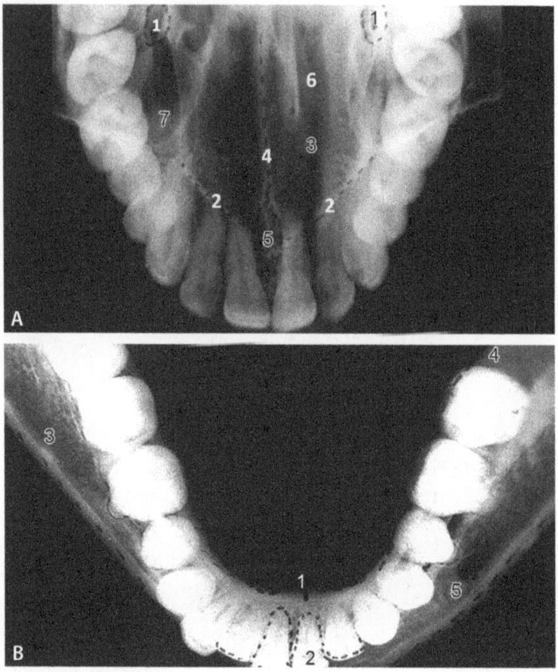

Figs 5.22A and B: True occlusal view. (A) Maxilla; 1. Nasolacrimal canal, 2. Lateral wall of the nasal fossa, 3. Nasal fossa, 4. Nasal septum, 5. Anterior nasal spine, 6. Inferior turbinate, 7. Maxillary antrum; (B) Mandible; 1. Genial tubercle, 2. Mandibular central incisors, 3. Buccal plate of mandibular body, 4. Mylohyoid ridge, 5. Mental foramen

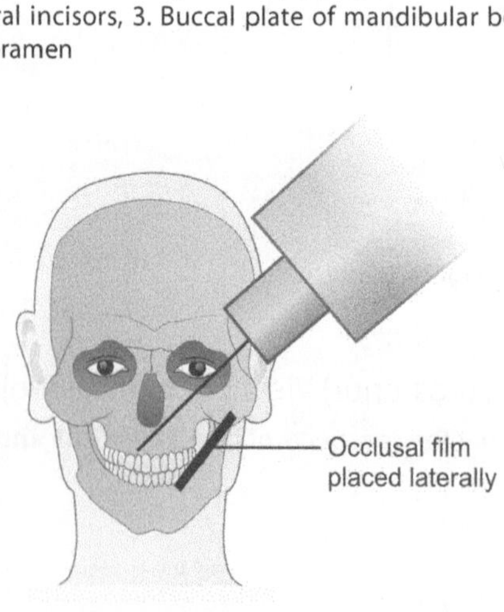

Fig. 5.23: Film and cone position for maxillary lateral occlusal projection

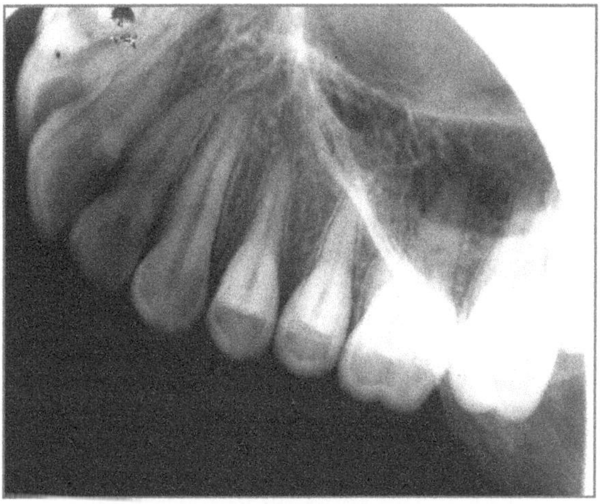

Fig. 5.24: Lateral maxillary occlusal view of jaw

Lateral Occlusal or Topographical View

This shows half of the alveolar ridge of (left or right side) maxilla or mandible **(Figs 5.23 and 5.24)**.

CHAPTER 6

X-ray Film Processing

When X-ray film is exposed to the information carrying X-ray beam or photons, photosensitive silver halide crystals in the film emulsion interact with these photons and get chemically changed. These chemically altered crystals are said to constitute the latent (Invisible) image on the film. While processing these latent images convert into manifest (visible) image.

When the silver halide crystals present in the film emulsion are irradiated, X-ray photons interact primarily with the bromide ion result in the removal of an electron from the bromide ions and converted into bromine atoms. The free electrons move through the crystal generating additional bromine atoms and recoil electron has sufficient kinetic energy to move about in crystal. When it strikes latent image site, it will impart negative charge to this region **(Fig. 6.1A)**. The positively charged free interstitial silver ions are attracted to the negatively charged latent image and become neutralized **(Figs 6.1B and C)** with the result that an atom of metallic silver is deposited at the latent image site. The larger the accumulation of silver atoms, the more sensitive the crystals.

Film processing: The primary actions of the processing solution is to convert the crystals with the latent images into black metallic silver grains that can be visualized and remove the unexposed silver bromide crystals **(Figs 6.2A to D)**.

There are two types of film processing:
1. Manual processing
2. Automatic processing

In manual processing, film processed by two methods:
1. Time temperature
2. Visual

Time temperature method (TT method): In this method, developing time is depends on the temperature of the developer solution. If the temperature of solution is high, it requires less developing time and vice versa.

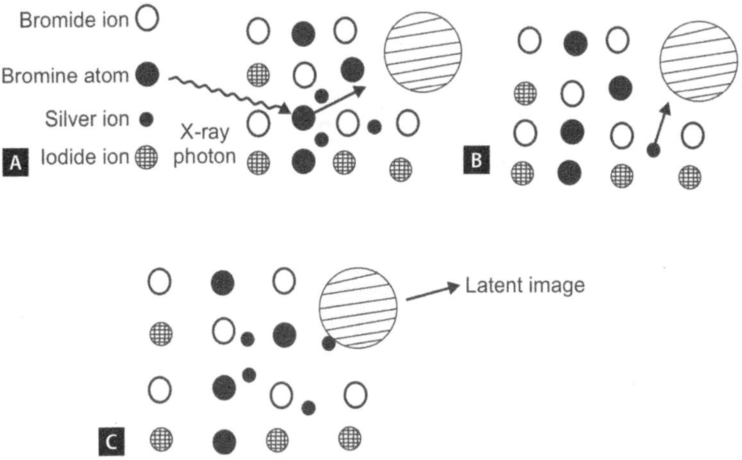

Figs 6.1A to C: Formation of the latent image. Before exposure of the film, a crystal contains silver, bromide, iodide ions, interstitial silver ions and latent image site. (A) During exposure X-ray photon interacts with the bromide ions and converted into bromine atoms and recoil electron have sufficient energy and they reach the latent image site and release all its negative charge to this site; (B) Positive charge of interstitial silver ions are attracted towards the negatively charged latent image site; (C) When the silver ions reach the site, they acquire an electron and become silver atoms, which constitute the latent image site. Developer causes conversion of these silver atoms into metallic silver

68°F	5 min
70°F	$4\frac{1}{2}$ min
72°F	4 min
76°F	3 min
80°F	$2\frac{1}{2}$ min

Visual method: In this method, films kept in developer solution until the high contrast of the image formation.

Film processing involves the following procedures:

- Immersion of exposed films in developer solution
- Rinsing in running water
- Immersion in fixing solution
- Film washing
- Drying and mounting for viewing

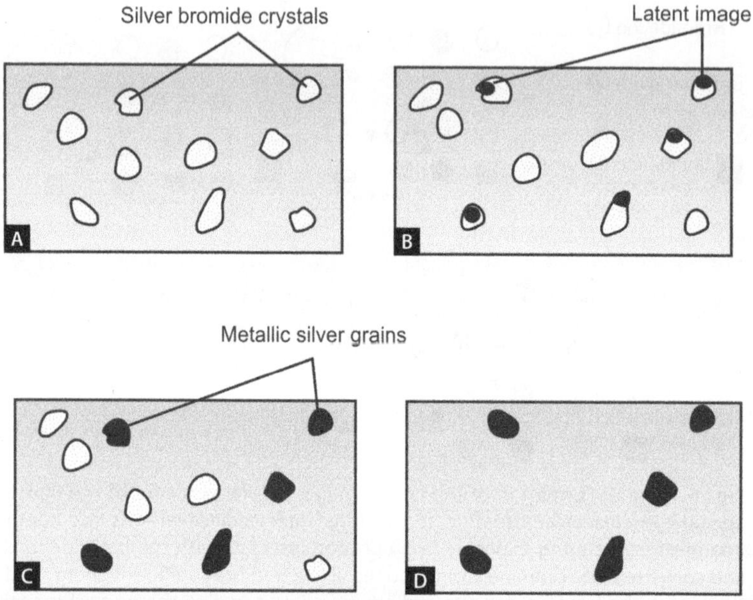

Figs 6.2A to D: Schematic diagram showing actions of processing solution on emulsion. (A) Before exposure, silver bromide crystals in the emulsion; (B) After exposure, latent image formation (shaded areas) on silver bromide crystals; (C) After development, latent image sites are converted into metallic silver; (D) After fixing, unexposed, undeveloped silver bromide crystals are dissolved and washed away by fixing solution retain only metallic silver

DEVELOPER SOLUTION

The action of the developer is to reduce all the silver ions in the exposed crystals to metallic silver. Developer solution contains four components:

1. Developer
2. Preservative
3. Activator
4. Restrainer

Developer

Primary function of the developing agent is to converting exposed silver halide crystals into metallic silver grains. Developer contains two main components.

1. *Elon* (Monomethyl-Para-amino-phenol sulfate)
2. *Hydroquinone* (Para-dihydroxy benzene).

Elon is less sensitive to temperature and brings out the gray shades in an image. Hydroquinone is more temperature sensitive and which inactive below 60°F and very active at above 70°F, thus temperature of the developing solution maintains at 60–70°F. This brings out the contrast of the image.

Preservative

Preservative used in developing solution is *sodium sulfite,* which has a great affinity for oxygen thus protects the developers from being oxidized by atmospheric oxygen.

Activator

The developers are only active at high pH values, i.e. above pH 11 (Alkali). This alkali serves as an activator (accelerator). Commonly used alkalis are:

- Sodium carbonate
- Sodium hydroxide
- Sodium metaborate
- Sodium tetraborate

Activator also serves to soften the gelatin so the developer agents can easily penetrate into the emulsion and reacts with the silver crystals.

Restrainer

Contains *potassium bromide.* Bromine is a product of the reduction of the silver halide crystals and the added bromide serves to depress the reduction by the unexposed crystals more than the exposed crystals and acts an anti-fog agent.

FIXING SOLUTION

The function of the fixing solution is to:

- Remove the undeveloped silver halide crystals from the emulsion. The presence of unexposed crystals cause film to be opaque and resultant radiograph is non-diagnostic.
- Which hardens the emulsion

Fixing solution contains four components:

1. Clearing agent
2. Acidifier
3. Preservative
4. Hardener

Clearing Agent

After development, unexposed silver halide crystals are cleared by dissolving and removing from the emulsion. Clearing agents contains *sodium or ammonium thiosulfate.*

Acidifier

Acetic acid is used to neutralize any contaminating alkali from the developing solution. If alkali and developing agents are not neutralized, then they causes developing of unexposed crystals and processing is continuing in the fixing tank result in fogging of the image.

Preservative

Sodium sulfite is used as a preservative. Its action is similar as in developer. It prevents the oxidation of any developer that may be carried on the films to fixer.

Hardener

- *Aluminum potassium sulfate*
- *Chromium potassium sulfate*

Which prevent damage to the gelatin by subsequent handling. It also shortens the drying time.

After fixing, film should be washed in a flow of water to remove all silver compounds, thiosulfate and its products. If not result in a sulfurizing of the image slowly which discolors the image and obscures diagnostic information this is because thiosulfate reacting with the silver to form brown silver sulfide **(Table 6.1)**.

Table 6.1: Summary of processing exposed X-ray film

Step 1	X-ray exposure	Latent image created
Step 2	Development	Converts latent image to black metallic silver
Step 3	Wash	Removes excess developer
Step 4	Fixing and Hardening	Dissolves out unexposed silver halide crystals and harden the emulsion
Step 5	Washing	Removes products of processing
Step 6	Dry	Removes water

FAULTY RADIOGRAPHS

Poor films result in loss of diagnostic information and loss of professional and patient time. The following is a list of common causes of faulty radiographs:

Light Radiographs

Causes

Processing errors:

- *Under developing radiographs* **(*Fig. 6.3*)**:
  - Low temperature of developer solution
  - Short time in developing
  - Inaccurate thermometer
- *Excessive fixation:*

  Corrections: Before processing of radiographs check for temperature of developing solution **(Table 6.2)** with thermometer, and adjust the developing and fixing time.

  If temperature of developing solution reaches above the maximum limit, then add ice blocks surrounding the processing tank to reduce the solution temperature. In case of lower temperature pour some hot water in the master tank that contains developing and fixing tank.
- Depleted developer solution
- Diluted or contaminated developer

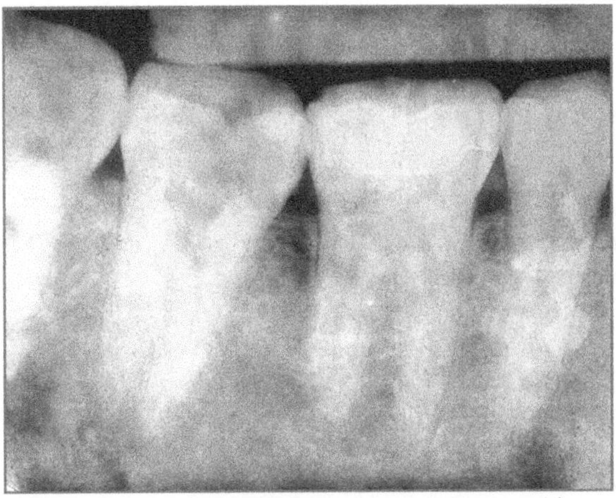

Fig. 6.3: Light radiograph

Table 6.2: Relation between temperature of developing solution and developing and fixing time

Temperature	*Developing time*	*Fixing time*
68°F	5 minutes	10 minutes
70°F	4½ minutes	9–10 minutes
72°F	4 minutes	8–9 minutes
76°F	3 minutes	6–7 minutes
80°F	2½ minutes	5–6 minutes

Corrections: Every 15 days change the developer and fixing solution to avoid depletion of solution which results in light radiographs. Cover the solution container so that contamination with other solution can be minimized.

Exposure Errors:
- Low mA
- Low kVp
- Less exposure time
- Increased film-target distance
- Reversed film packet positioning in the month.

Corrections: Proper selection of milliampere, kilovoltage and exposure time to avoid errors in radiographs.

Target to film distance is maintained 8 inch in bisecting angle and 12–16 inch in paralleling cone technique.

Check the front or tube side of the film packet is facing towards the X-ray cone.

Dark Radiographs

Causes

Processing Errors
- *Overdeveloping* **(*Fig. 6.4*)**:
  - High temperature of developer
  - Long time in developer
- *High concentration of developer*
- *Under fixing:*

  Corrections: Adjust the temperature and time of developing and fixing as discussed earlier. If the concentration of developer solution is high, add water to make dilute.
- Accidental exposure to light

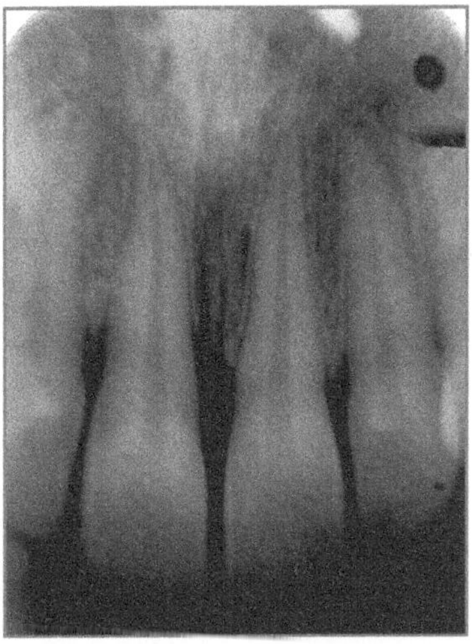

Fig. 6.4: Dark radiograph

- *Improper safe lighting:*
  Corrections: While processing makes sure that no light leakage in to the room. Unwrap the film packet in dark room only to avoid accidental exposure of light causing dark radiographs.

Adopt proper safe light. Safe light should be orange or red color only because these colors have longer wavelength does not affect on the light sensitive silver halide crystals. Safe light bulb should not be more than 15 watts, and it should be covered with GBX filter. Working surface should be 4 feet from the safe light.

Exposure Errors:

- High mA
- High kVp
- More Exposure time
- Decreased Film-target distance.

Corrections:

- Proper selection of Milliamperage, kilovolts and exposure time without alteration in the density and contrast of the radiographs.
- Adjust the film target distance without any effect on the density of the image by altering the mA, kVp and exposure time.

Insufficient Contrast

Causes

- Underdeveloped
- Under exposure
- Low kVp
- Excessive film fog.

Corrections:

- Fix the developing time according to temperature of developer.
- Lower the kVp and exposure time results in high contrast and reduce the film fog.

Film Fog (Fig. 6.5)

Causes

- *Improper safe light:*
  - Improper filter
  - Excessive bulb wattage
  - Inadequate distance between bulb and working surface
  - Prolonged exposure to safe light
  - Cracked safe light filter.

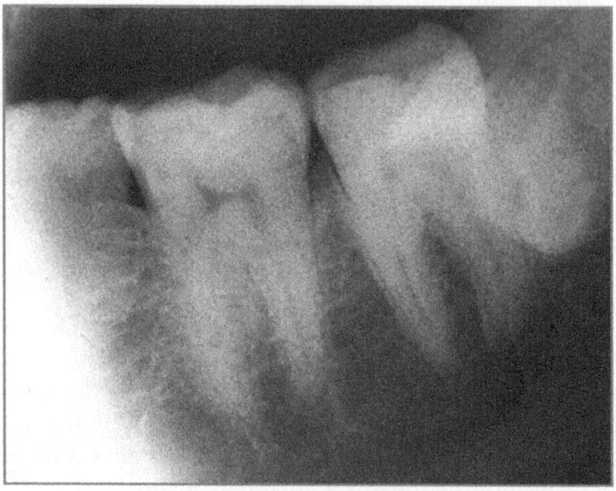

Fig. 6.5: Fogged radiograph

Corrections:
- Check the proper function of safe light.
- Working surface should be 4 feet away from the safe light.
- If any crack in the filter, immediately replace with new one.

- Over developing:
- Contaminated solution
- *Deteriorated film:*
  - Stored at high temperature
  - Stored at high humidity
  - Exposed to irradiation
  - Outdated

Corrections:
- Adjust the developing time.
- Cover the processor container to avoid contamination with other solution .
- Outdated films should not be used.
- Films should be placed in dark, cool, dry and protected from light streak or X-ray beam.

Dark Spots or Lines on Radiographs

Causes

- Finger print contamination
- Film contaminated with developer before processing
- Excessive bending of films
- Film in contact with tank or another film during fixing.

Corrections:
- Wash and dry hands thoroughly before processing films.
- Avoid contaminating the hands.
- Handle the films by the edges only.
- Working surface should be clean and free from developer solution.
- Should not be bend the film excessively while placing X-ray film in to the mouth.
- Separate films so that no contact takes place during fixing.

Light Spots or Lines on Radiographs

Causes

- Film contaminated with fixer before processing
- Film in contact with tank or another film during developing.

Corrections:
- Use clean working surface in dark room.
- Separate the film in developer tank.

Yellow or Brown Stains on Radiographs (Fig. 6.6)

Causes

- Depleted developer
- Depleted fixer
- Insufficient washing
- Contaminated solution

Corrections:
- Change the developer and fixer solutions every 15 days.
- Wash the film properly in water at least for 10–15 min after fixing to remove the residual fixing solution which results in yellow or brown stains after a few days.
- Avoid contamination between each solution.

Blurred Radiographs

Causes

- Movement of patient
- Movement of X-ray tubes
- Double exposure

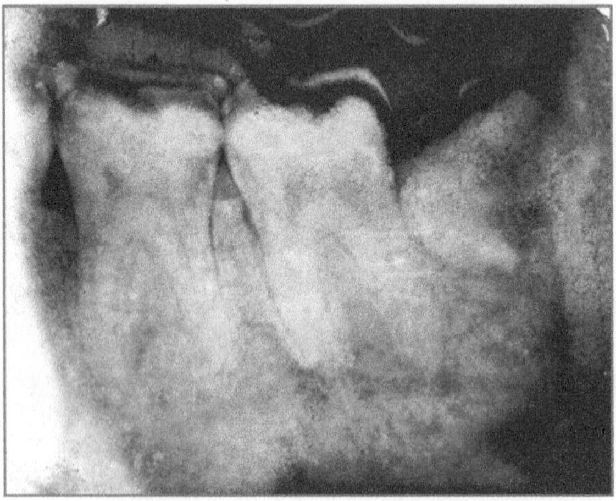

Fig. 6.6: Brown stain over the radiograph

Corrections:

- Stabilize the patient and X-ray cone while exposure.
- Care should be taken to separate exposed and unexposed X-ray films to avoid accidental re-exposure of films.

Cone Cut (Fig. 6.7)

Causes

- Improper placement of film
- Improper placement of X-ray cone.

Corrections:

- Proper positioning of X-ray film in such a way that, center of X-ray film should contact with the interesting tooth.
- Make certain that the X-ray beam is centered over the film.

Dimensional Changes

Causes

- Elongated image **(Fig. 6.8)**
- Foreshortened image **(Fig. 6.9)**
- Superimposition/overlapping.

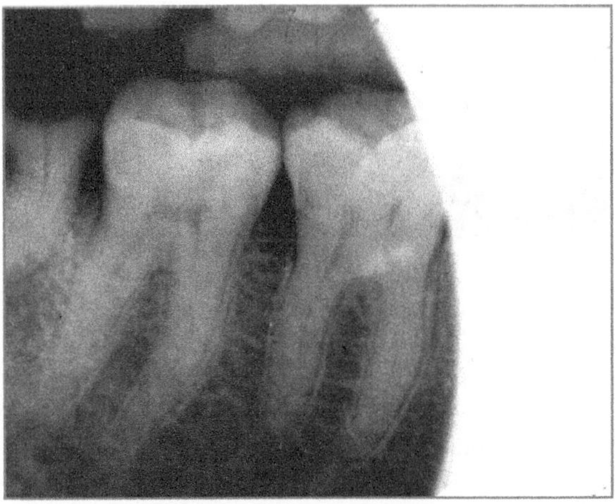

Fig. 6.7: Radiograph showing cone cut

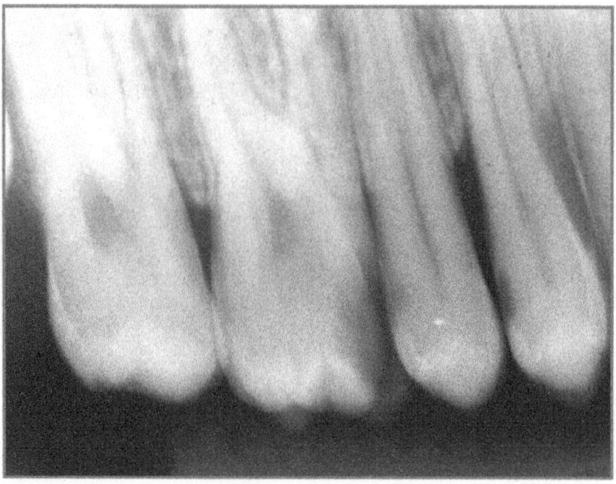

Fig. 6.8: Elongated image

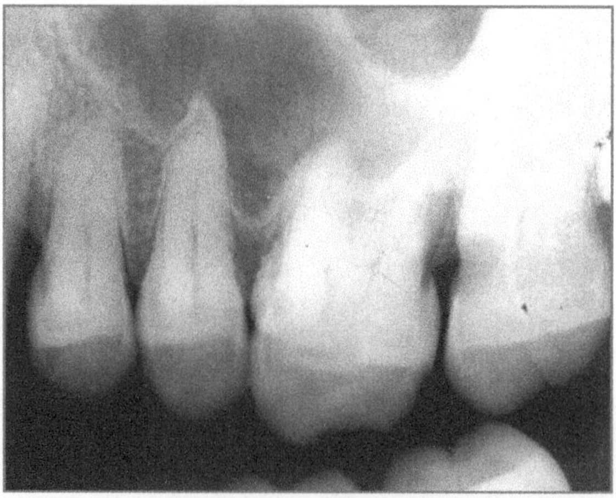

Fig. 6.9: Shortened image

Corrections:

- More vertical angulation of X-ray tube results in foreshortening of image.
- Less vertical angulation causes elongation of image.
- Improper horizontal angulation results in overlapping or superimposition of image.

Scratched Film (Fig. 6.10)

Causes

Soft film emulsion is removed from the sharp object or film hanger during processing.

Corrections:

- Care should be taken while placing a film with hanger in the processing solutions.
- Avoid contact with the other film hangers during processing.

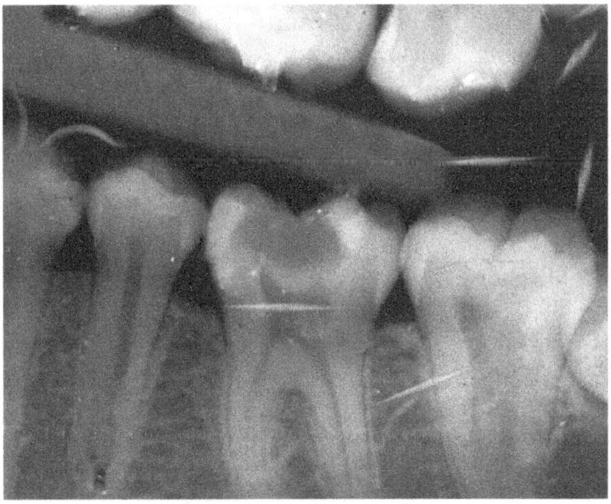

Fig. 6.10: Scratched film

CHAPTER 7

Normal Radiographic Anatomy

The radiographic recognition of disease requires a sound knowledge of the radiographic appearance of normal structures. Most patients show many of the normal radiographic landmarks, but it is a rare patient who shows them all.

There are many normal anatomical landmarks, both radiolucent and radiopaque in maxilla and mandible.

RADIOLUCENT LANDMARKS OF MAXILLA

- Tooth—Pulp
- Periodontal structures—Periodontal ligament space, bone marrow spaces
- Incisive foramen
- Intermaxillary suture
- Nasal fossa
- Nasopalatine canal
- Lateral fossa
- Nasolacrimal canal
- Maxillary sinus.

Tooth

Pulp in normal tooth is composed of soft tissue appears radiographically as radiolucent.

Diffuse radiolucent areas with ill-defined borders may be appear radiographically on the mesial or distal aspects of tooth in the cervical regions between the edge of the enamel and the crest of the alveolar ridge, this phenomenon called *"Cervical burnout"* this radiolucent results from the contrast with the adjacent radiopaque enamel and alveolar bone and decreased X-ray absorption.

Periodontal Structures

Periodontal ligament is composed of collagen and appears as a radiolucent space between lamina dura and the root. The width of periodontal space varies with the tooth and location around the tooth. It is thinner in the middle 1/3rd and wider in cervical 1/3rd and root apex. Bone marrow spaces are small and numerous in anterior and larger in posterior.

Incisive Foramen or Nasopalatine or Anterior Palatine Foramen

It is the oral terminus of the nasopalatine canal, which transmits nasopalatine nerves. Radiographically image is appears as oval or round-shaped radiolucent usually projected between the middle and apical 1/3rd of the roots of the central incisors **(Figs 7.1 and 7.2)**. It is important because it is a potential site of cyst formation.

Intermaxillary Suture

This appears between two portions of the premaxilla as a thin radiolucent line between the centers of incisors root and extending from the crest of the alveolar bone to the posterior aspect of the palatal borders. It is lined by cortical bone, which appears as a radiopaque **(Figs 7.1 and 7.3)**.

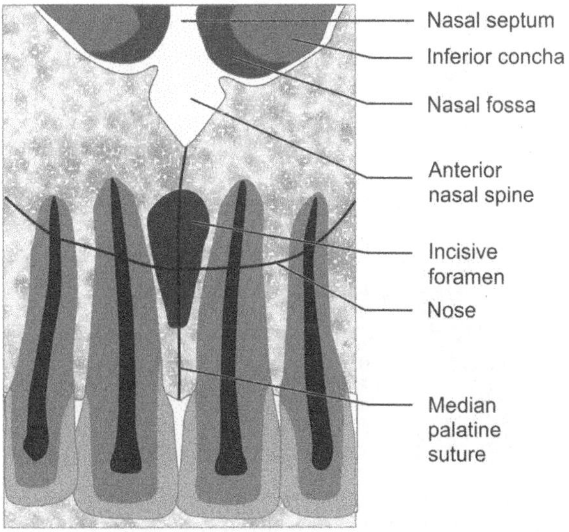

Fig. 7.1: Schematic representation of anatomical landmarks in maxilla

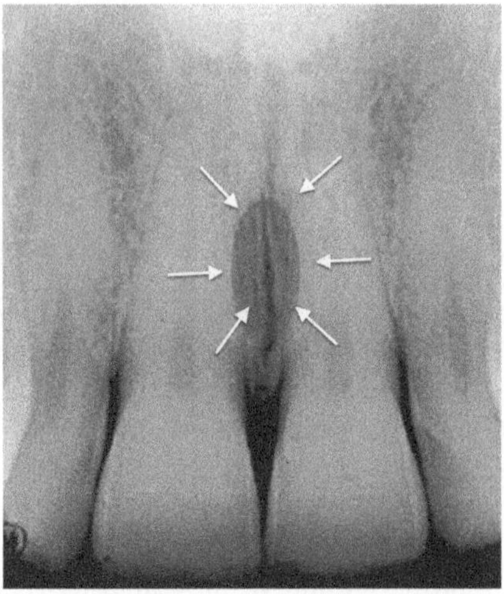

Fig. 7.2: Radiograph of maxillary incisors showing oval-shaped radiolucency between central incisors

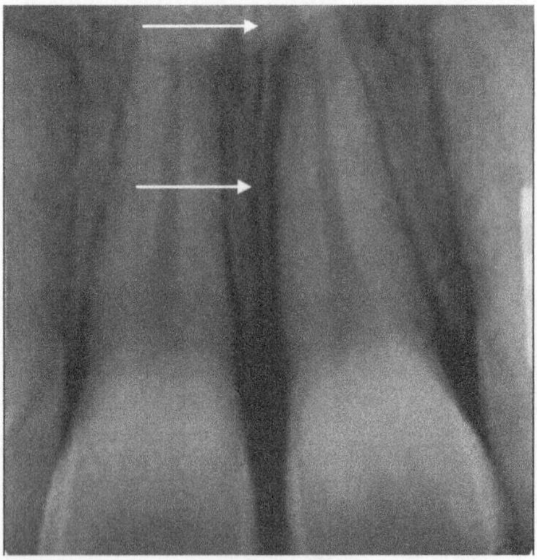

Fig. 7.3: Radiograph of maxillary incisors showing thin radiolucent line (arrows) with radiopaque border begins from alveolar crest run posteriorly between central incisors

Nasal Fossa

Air filled nasal fossa lies just above the oral cavity appears radiolucent on intraoral periapical radiograph of maxillary anterior teeth **(Fig. 7.1)**. Nasal septum, a radiopaque line divides the two fossa. The margins of the fossa are lined with compact bone appears radiographically as a radiopaque line **(Fig. 7.4)** and posterior limit of nasal fossa can be seen at 1st molar region on periapical radiographs.

Nasopalatine Canal

This is usually not seen in periapical film but also viewed on occlusal films. This canal originates at two foramina at the floor of the nasal cavity. The opening are on either side of the nasal septum appears as a radiolucent.

Lateral Fossa

Lateral fossa is slight depression in the maxilla near the apex of the lateral incisor **(Fig. 7.5A)**. On periapical radiograph this region appears as diffuse radiolucent **(Fig. 7.5B)**. The image is misinterpreted as periapical pathology unless examined for intact lamina dura and absence of clinical symptoms.

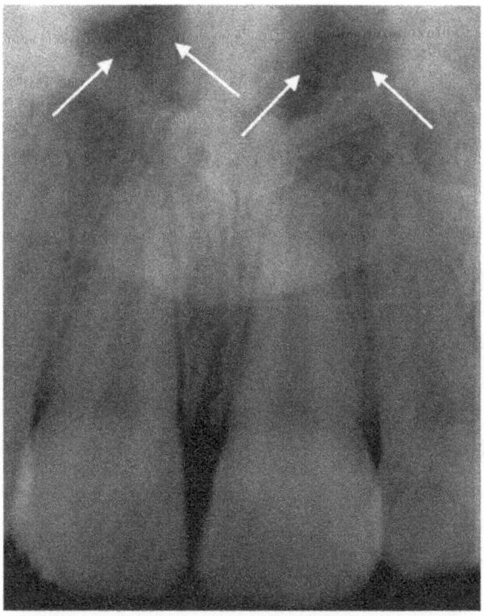

Fig. 7.4: Maxillary anterior radiograph showing nasal fossa on either side of nasal septum (arrows)

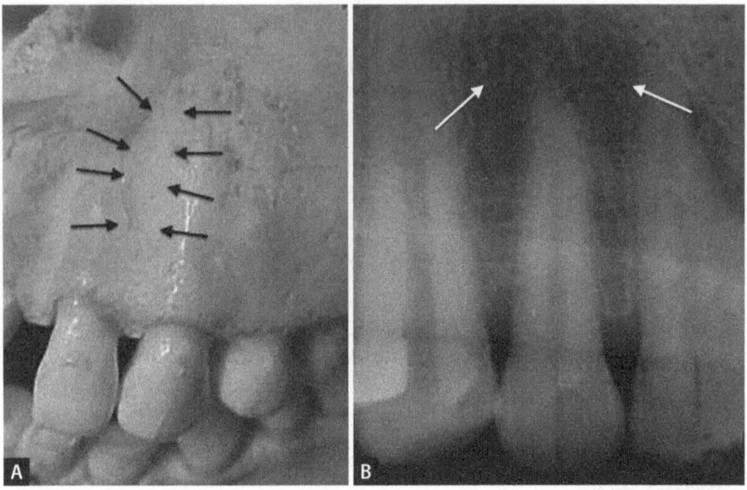

Figs 7.5A and B: (A) Lateral fossa appeared as gentle depression at the apex or between lateral incisor and cuspid on maxillary bone (arrows); (B) Maxillary anterior radiograph showing diffuse radiolucent at apex of the lateral incisor (arrows)

Nasolacrimal Canal

This is seen in occlusal films as a round or oval-shaped radiolucent area over the roots of the maxillary first molar.

Maxillary Sinus

It appears as dark shadows over the posterior tooth usually from premolar to the tuberosity region. On intraoral periapical radiograph it appears as the either U-shaped or W-shaped radiolucency with radiopaque septa in between it **(Fig. 7.6)**.

RADIOPAQUE LANDMARKS OF MAXILLA

- Tooth—enamel, dentine,
- Periodontal structures—cementum, lamina dura and trabeculae
- Anterior nasal spine
- Nasal septum
- Inferior concha
- Nasolabial fold
- Y line of Ennis

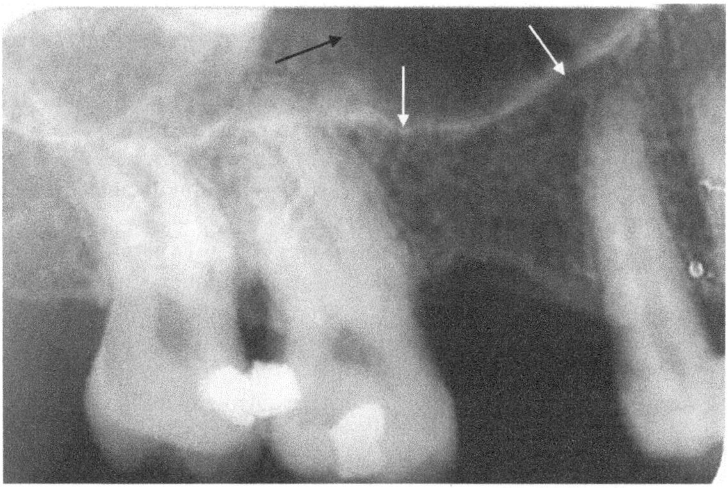

Fig. 7.6: Maxillary posterior radiograph showing maxillary sinus, floor wall (white arrows) and septa in between (black arrow)

- Zygomatic process of maxilla
- Maxillary tuberosity
- Coronoid process of mandible
- Pterygoid plates
- Hamular process.

Tooth

Enamel, dentine and cementum are denser material appears radiographically as a radiopaque.

Periodontal Structures

Lamina dura is a radiographic terminology, which runs from the crest of the alveolar bone along the root of the tooth. Anatomically it is the edge of the cortical bone.

It is important in diagnosis of certain periapical infections. The presence of an intact lamina dura around the apex of the tooth suggests a vital pulp.

Cancellous bone (Trabecular bone or spongiosa): Lies between the cortical plates in both Jaws. This contains radiopaque trabecular network surrounding many radiolucent pockets of bone marrow. Trabeculae are arranged in irregular pattern in maxilla. Trabeculae does not allow X-ray to pass through it and appeared as radiopaque, but marrow spaces appeared radiolucent because X-ray can easily pass through it.

- *Anterior maxilla:* Trabeculae are thin and numerous forming fine trabecular network. Marrow spaces in anterior maxilla are small and numerous.
- *Posterior maxilla:* Marrow spaces are larger and trabeculae pattern is similar to that in the anterior maxilla.
- *Anterior mandible:* Trabeculae are thick and course pattern arranged as horizontally oriented but they are few in number. Marrow spaces are larger and few in number.
- *Posterior mandible:* Trabeculae are arranged as step ladder like pattern and marrow spaces are large.

Alterations in the trabecular pattern or marrow spaces suggestive of pathology.

Anterior Nasal Spine

It lies below the junction of the inferior end of the nasal septum and the inferior outline of the nasal fossa. It is radiopaque because of its bony spicules usually *v* shaped **(Figs 7.7A and B)**.

Nasal Septum

It is vertical bony wall that divides nasal cavity and nasal fossa into left and right **(Fig. 7.8A)**. On periapical radiograph of maxillary central incisors, nasal septum appears as thick radiopaque line above the root apex of central incisors, which divides nasal fossa into left and right halves **(Fig. 7.8B)**.

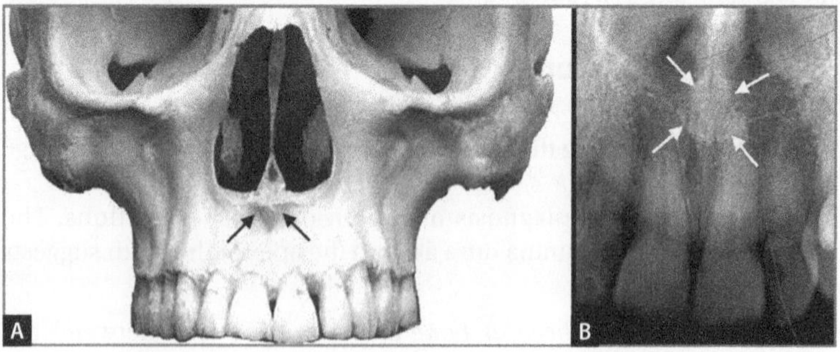

Figs 7.7A and B: (A) Spike-shaped nasal septum; (B) Thick radiopacity seen at the junction of nasal fossa and the nasal septum (arrows)

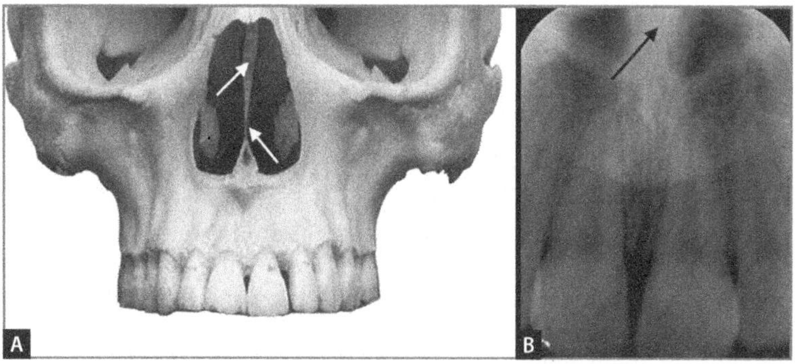

Figs 7.8A and B: (A) Nasal septum a vertical bony wall divides left and right nasal cavity (white arrows); (B) Maxillary central radiograph shows vertical radiopaque portion that divides nasal fossa into left and right (black arrow)

Inferior Concha

The nasal cavity contains three concha namely superior, middle and inferior concha **(Fig. 7.9A)**, but on periapical radiograph of maxillary incisors shows only inferior concha as a radiopaque shadow extending from the lateral wall of nasal cavity for varying distance towards the nasal septum **(Fig. 7.9B)**. The appearance of inferior concha on periapical radiograph depends on the position of X-ray film, X-ray cone and the vertical angulation of cone placement.

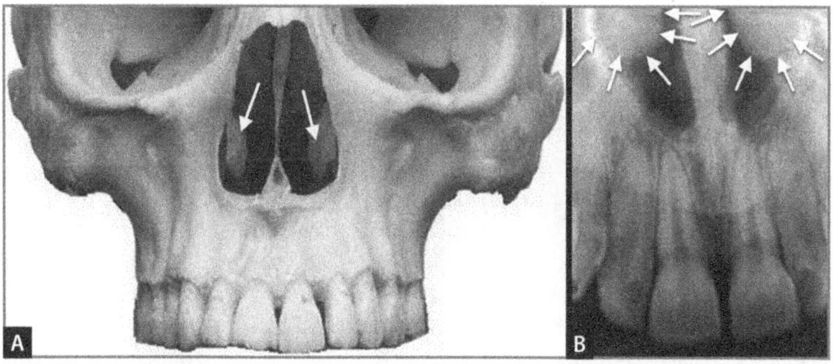

Figs 7.9A and B: (A) Inferior concha of the nasal cavity (white arrows); (B) Maxillary central incisors radiograph revealed radiopaque shadow on either side of the nasal septum (white arrows)

Nasolabial Fold

Periapical radiographs of the canine premolar region are frequently traversed by a radiopaque oblique line. It is the thick cheek tissue superimposed on the tooth and the alveolar process.

Y Line of Ennis (Inverted Y)

Y line of Ennis is not a true anatomical landmark but seen only on periapical radiographs due to superimposition of the floor of the nasal cavity (straight radiopaque line) and the border of the maxillary sinus (curved radiopaque line).

On radiographically, Y line of Ennis found superior to the maxillary canine apex. Sometimes it will be more distal and superior to the first premolar apices. It is commonly found at the junction of posterior region of nasal fossa and anterior aspect of maxillary antrum as inverted Y line, where straight horizontal line is the border of nasal fossa and the curved line perpendicular to the horizontal line refers to the anterior margin of antrum. Y line of Ennis is well-defined with corticated border and appeared as inverted Y shape **(Fig. 7.10)**.

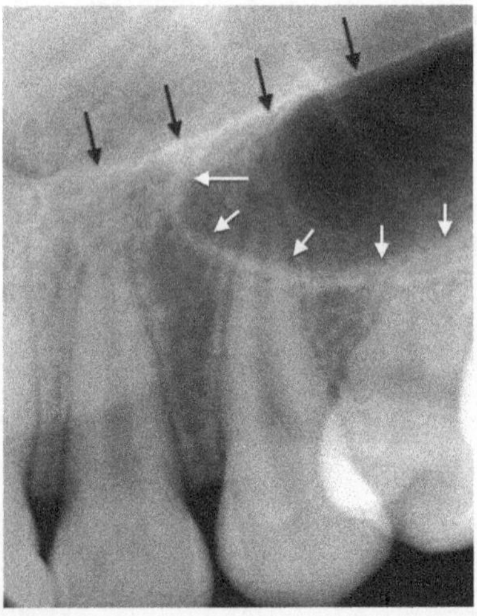

Fig. 7.10: Maxillary radiograph of canine shows junction of posterior limit of nasal fossa (black arrows) and anterior part of maxillary antrum (white arrows)

Zygomatic Process of Maxilla

On periapical radiograph, the zygomatic process appears as a thick *U*- or *V*-shaped radiopaque line **(Fig. 7.11)** above the maxillary sinus. The position and shape of zygomatic process depends on the high position of X-ray cone placement and vertical angulation of X-ray cone.

Maxillary Tuberosity

The maxillary tuberosity is a rounded prominence of bone that extends posterior to the third molar region **(Fig. 7.12A)**. On periapical radiograph, it appears as a radiopaque bulge distal to the third molar area **(Fig. 7.12B)**.

Coronoid Process of Mandible

Coronoid process of the mandible is frequently apparent on periapical radiographs of maxillary molar region superimposed over the maxillary tuberosity as a triangular radiopacity **(Fig. 7.13)**.

Pterygoid Plates

The medial and lateral pterygoid plate lies immediately posterior to the tuberosity of the maxilla **(Fig. 7.14A)**. It appears as a single homogeneous radiopaque shadow without any evidence of trabeculation **(Fig. 7.14B)**.

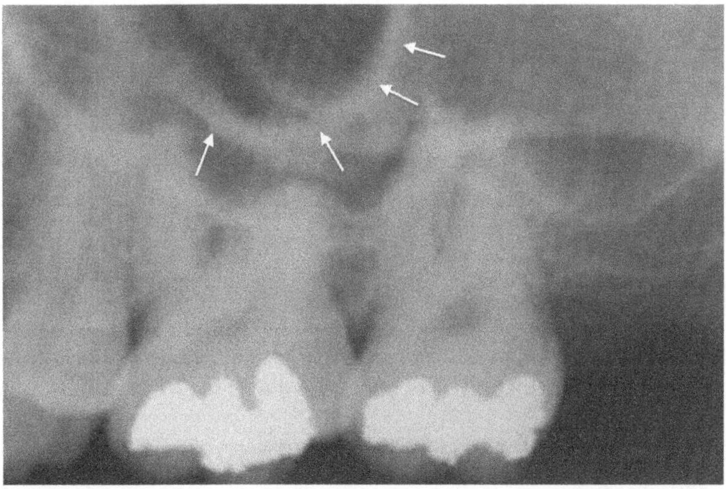

Fig. 7.11: Maxillary molar radiograph shows thick U-shaped radiopaque structure just above the maxillary antrum (arrows)

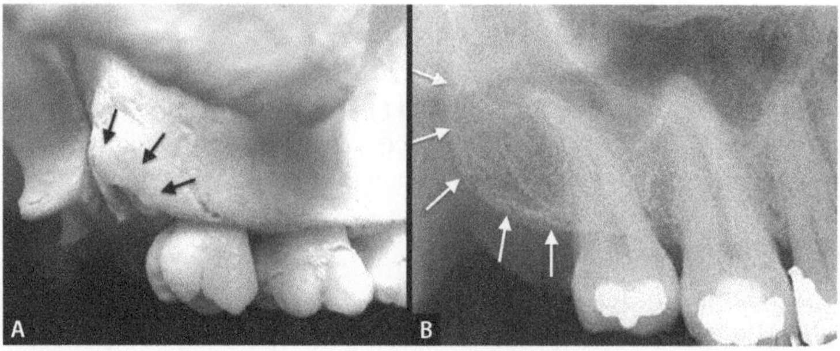

Figs 7.12A and B: (A) Maxillary tuberosity position distal to the third molar (black arrows); (B) On radiograph, it appeared as radiopaque prominence distal to the third molar (white arrows)

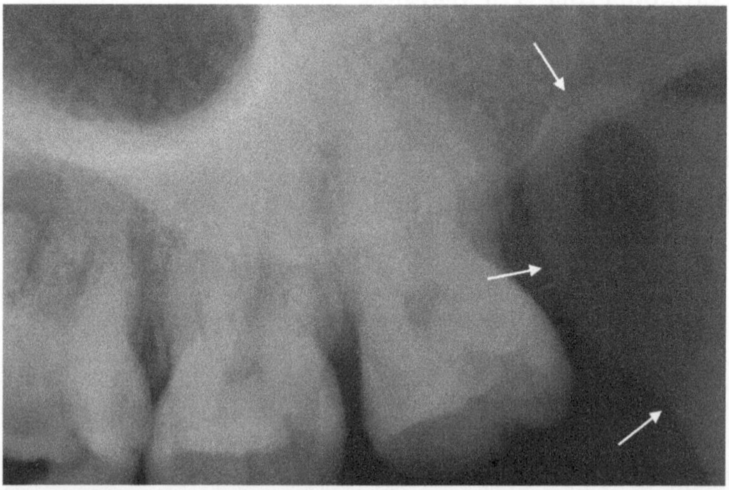

Fig. 7.13: Maxillary molar radiography revealed radiopaque coronoid process of mandible at distal to the third molar

Hamular Process

It is small hook like projection of the bone extending downward from the medial pterygoid plate of sphenoid bone distal to the tuberosity and shows some trabeculation on detail evaluation **(Figs 7.14A and B)**.

RADIOLUCENT LANDMARKS OF MANDIBLE

- Tooth—Pulp
- Periodontal structures—Periodontal ligament space, bone marrow spaces

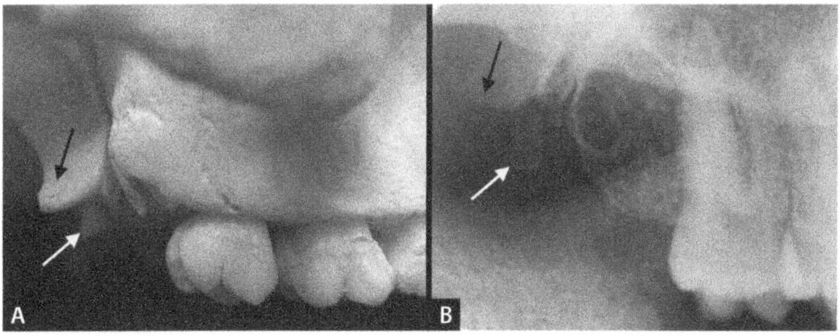

Figs 7.14A and B: (A) Pterygoid plate (black arrow) and hamular process (white arrow); (B) Maxillary distal to the third molar radiograph revealed hamular process and pterygoid plate

- Symphysis
- Lingual foramen
- Mental fossa
- Mental Foramen
- Mandibular canal
- Submandibular gland fossa.

Tooth

Pulp appears as a radiolucent because it contains connective tissue.

Periodontal Structures

Bone marrow spaces are larger in mandible.

Symphysis

Radiographs of infants in mandibular symphysal region shows radiolucent line in the midline of the jaw. This suture fuses at the end of first year of life. After which it is no longer evident on radiographically.

Lingual Foramen

A periapical radiograph of mandibular anterior region demonstrates a small radiolucent dot surrounded by the cortical wall which terminates the incisive branch of the mandibular canal **(Figs 7.15 and 7.16)**.

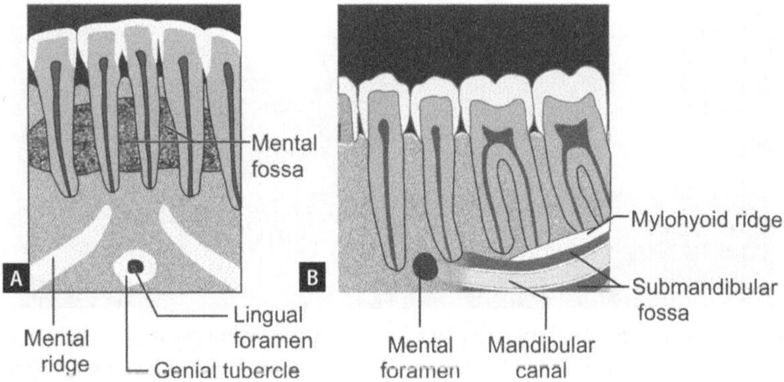

Figs 7.15A and B: (A) Schematic representation of anatomical landmarks of mandibular anterior region; (B) Anatomical landmarks of mandibular posterior region

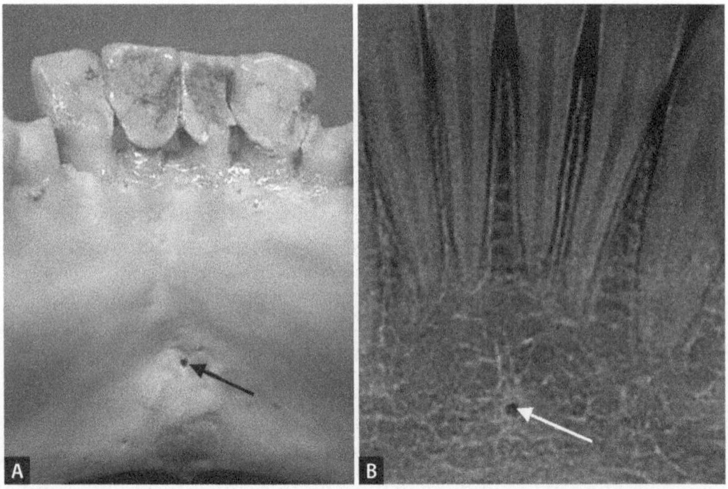

Figs 7.16A and B: (A) Lingual aspect of midline of mandible showing small round openings known as lingual foramen; (B) Mandibular anterior radiograph showing lingual foramen

Mental Fossa

It is a depression on the labial aspect of the mandible **(Fig. 7.17A)**, which appears radiographically as a diffuse radiolucent on anterior surface of mandible between alveolar ridge and mental ridge **(Figs 7.17A and 7.17B)**.

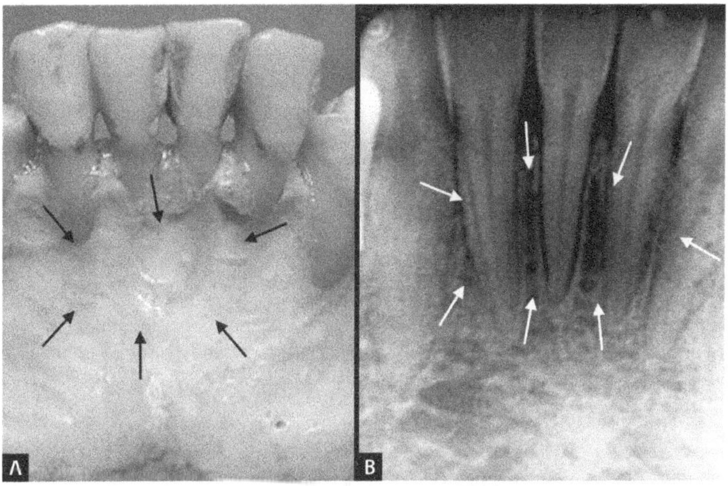

Figs 7.17A and B: (A) Depression over the labial aspect of the midline of the mandible above the mental ridge; (B) Diffuse radiolucent on mandibular incisors at apex mimics periapical pathology

Mental Foramen

It is a small ovoid or round radiolucent area located in the apical region of the mandibular premolars and it is the anterior end of the mandibular canal through which blood vessels and nerves supply to the lower anterior regions.

Radiographically appeared as a small ovoid or round radiolucent area located in the apical region of the mandibular second premolar. When mental foramen projected over the premolar apices, it may mimic the periapical pathology. In such cases, presence of lamina dura determines the true nature of the disease or shift cone technique revealed the exact nature of the radiolucent structure **(Figs 7.15B and 7.18)**.

Mandibular Canal

Mandibular canal extends from the mandibular foramen located near the middle of the ramus to mental foramen anteriorly **(Fig. 7.19A)**. Radiographically canal is a dark linear shadow with thin radiopaque superior and inferior borders. Which runs just inferior to the apices of the posteriorly teeth **(Fig. 7.19B)**.

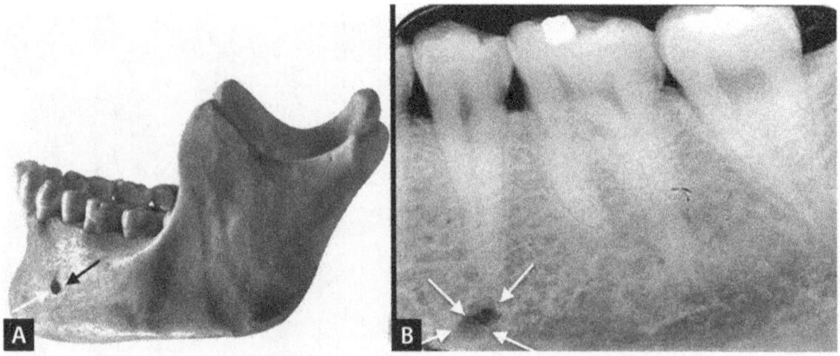

Figs 7.18A and B: (A) Mental foramen lies halfway between alveolar crest and lower border of mandible; (B) On radiograph, round- or oval-shaped radiolucent at the apex of mandibular second premolar

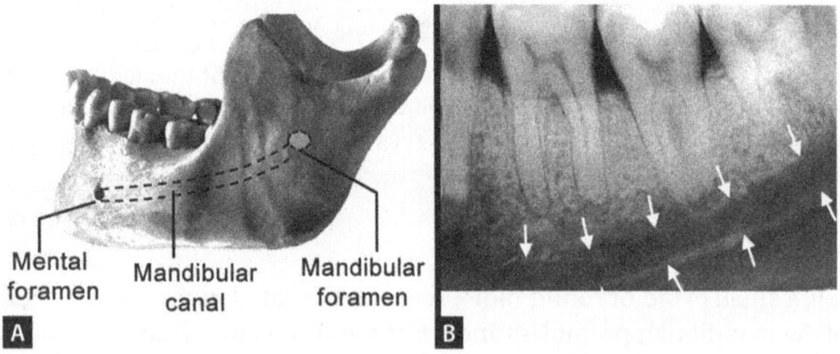

Figs 7.19A and B: (A) Mandibular canal origin at mandibular foramen on lingual aspect of ramus of mandible runs downward and forward and opens at mental foramen near the premolar teeth; (B) On periapical radiograph, appeared as radiolucent canal with corticated (radiopaque) border

Submandibular Gland Fossa

On the lingual surface of mandibular body immediately below the mylohyoid ridge in the molar area, there is depression in the bone, which accommodates the submandibular gland **(Fig. 7.20A)** and appears radiographically as diffuse radiolucent area, mimics the periapical infection **(Fig. 7.20B)**.

RADIOPAQUE LANDMARKS OF MANDIBLE

- Tooth—Enamel and dentine
- Periodontal structures—Cementum, lamina dura, alveolar crest, and trabecular pattern

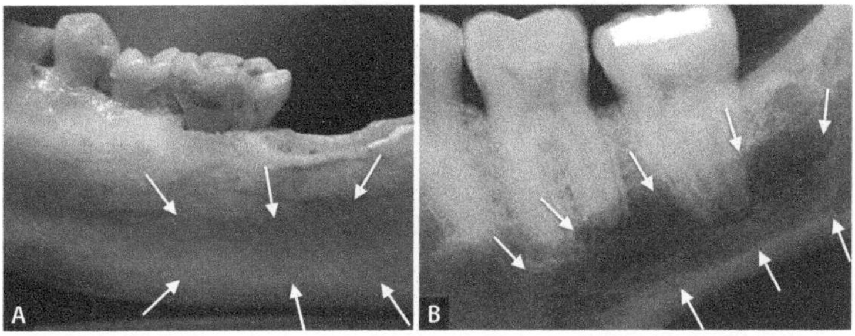

Figs 7.20A and B: (A) Depression on lingual surface of body of the mandible just below the mylohyoid ridge; (B) Submandibular gland fossa appeared as large radiolucent area at the apices of mandibular posterior teeth

- Genial tubercle
- Mental ridge
- Mylohyoid ridge
- External oblique ridge
- Inferior border of the mandible.

Tooth

Enamel and dentin appears as radiopaque.

Periodontal Structures

Cementum, alveolar bone and cementum appear as radiopaque.

Genial Tubercle (Mental Spine)

It is located on the lingual surface of the anterior mandible as a bony protuberance with spine shaped **(Fig. 7.21A)**. They serve to attach genioglossal and geniohyoid muscles to the mandible. In periapical radiographs, radiopaque mass in the midline below the incisors root **(Fig. 7.21B)**. This appeared well on occlusal radiograph as a radiopaque projection **(Fig. 7.21C)**.

Mental Ridge

Mental ridge represent the raised portions of the mental protuberance on either side of the midline **(Fig. 7.22A)**. On periapical radiographs of the mandibular central incisors shows radiopaque lines runs bilaterally forward and upward toward the middle **(Fig. 7.22B)**.

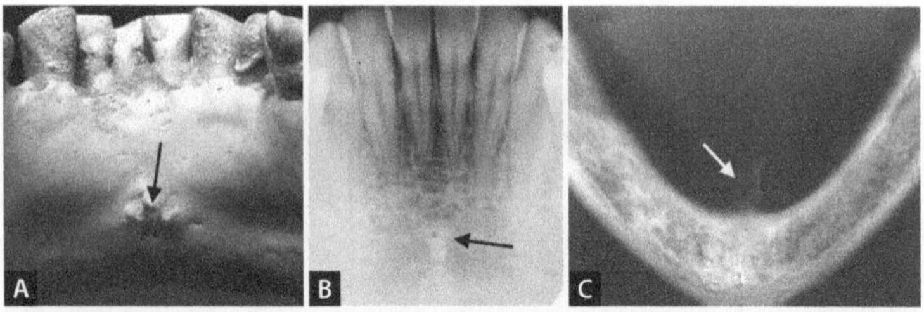

Figs 7.21A to C: (A) Genial tubercle is spike like projection on lingual surface of the midline of the mandible; (B) Radiopaque mass apparent on periapical radiograph; (C) Genial tubercle is very much evident on occlusal radiograph

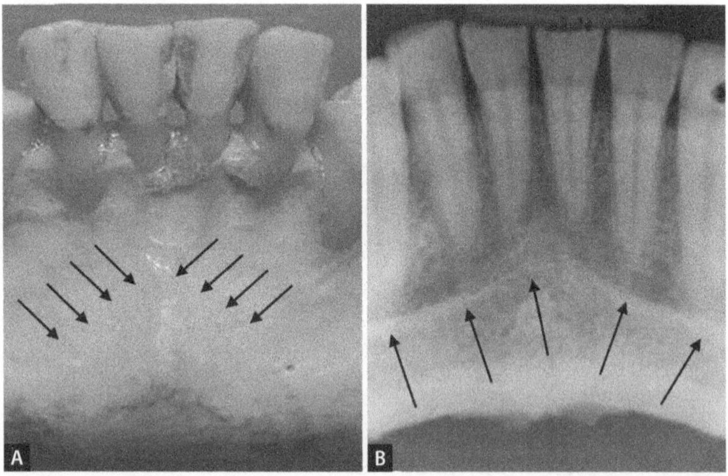

Figs 7.22A and B: (A) Mental ridge appears as protuberance on either side of the midline (arrows) of labial aspect of the mandible; (B) Mental ridge on the facial aspect of mandible appear as radiopaque ridge on radiograph

Mylohyoid Ridge

It is slightly irregular bone on the lingual surface of body of mandible **(Fig. 7.23A)**. Extending from the area of the 3rd molar to the premolar region, this serves as an attachment for the mylohyoid muscle. Periapical radiographs shows, diffuse radiopaque line along the apices of mandible posterior tooth **(Fig. 7.23B)**.

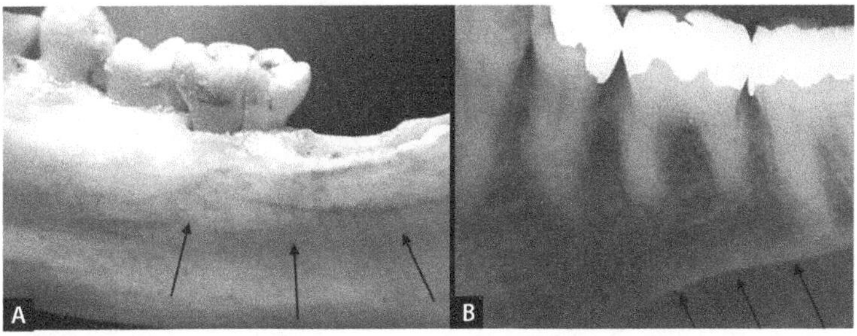

Figs 7.23A and B: (A) Mylohyoid ridge on the lingual surface of mandibular bone; (B) Diffuse radiopaque line at the molar apices

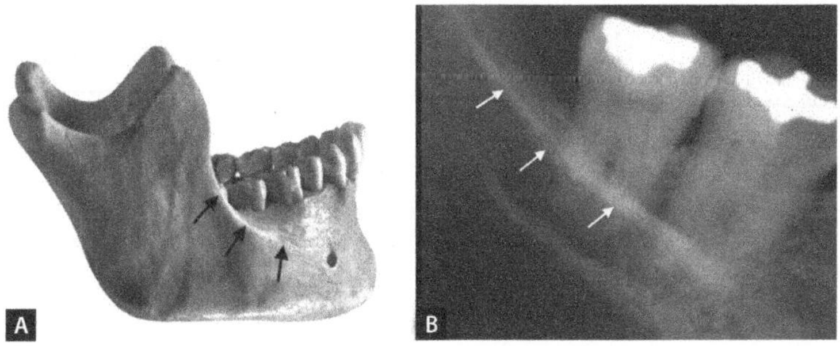

Figs 7.24A and B: (A) External oblique ridge is a bony elevation runs from anterior border of ramus (arrows); (B) A linear radiopaque along the roots of the molar teeth (arrows)

External Oblique Ridge

It is the continuation of the anterior border of the mandibular ramus runs along the lateral to the alveolar process up to 1st molar. The bony elevation gradually flattens **(Fig. 7.24A)**. This serves as an attachment of the buccinator muscle. In periapical radiograph, it is evident as a radiopaque line of varying width appeared above the mylohyoid ridge **(Fig. 7.24B)**.

Inferior Border of the Mandible

Occasionally inferior border of mandible will be seen on periapical radiograph as a dense, broad radiopaque band of bone **(Fig. 7.25)**.

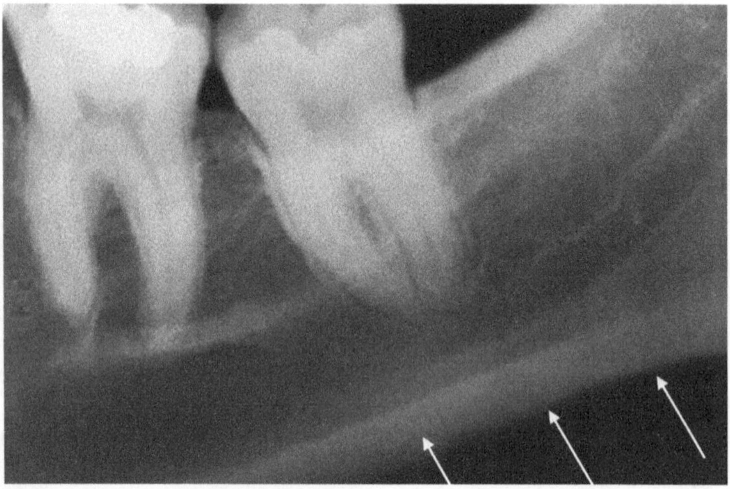

Fig. 7.25: Lower border of mandible appears as dense corticated radiopaque band

Table 7.1: Radiographic appearance of some restorative materials

Radiopaque	*Radiolucent*
• Stainless steel pins	• Silicate restorations
• Base material	• Porcelain
• Gutta-percha	• Composite restoration
• Silver points	
• Stainless steel crowns	
• Orthodontic appliances	

Radiographic appearance of some restorative materials is tabulated in **Table 7.1**.

CHAPTER

8 Extraoral Radiography

EXTRAORAL X-RAY FILM OR SCREEN FILM (INDIRECT EXPOSURE FILM)

Screen film or extraoral films are mainly used in combination with intensifying screens for extraoral radiographs such as panoramic, cephalometric and skull radiographs.

Extraoral film also called indirect exposure because X-ray photons strikes the intensifying screens, then these intensifying screen emits visible light exposes the X-ray film indirectly.

Basic composition of extra- and intraoral films are similar, but in extraoral, dyes are added to emulsion specifically increases the absorption of the wavelength of the specific visible light emit by the intensifying screen, hence extraoral films are sensitive primarily to visible light rather than X-ray photons.

It is important to use the appropriate screen film combination recommended by the screen or film manufacturer so that emission and absorption characteristics of the screen and films are matched. Some screen films are sensitive to blue light (*Kodak X-Omat* and *Ektamat films*), whereas others have sensitive to green visible light (*Kodak Ortho* and *T-Mat films*). Different emulsions are manufactured which are sensitive to the different colors of light emitted by different types of intensifying screens. They are:

- Standard silver halide emulsion—sensitive to *BLUE* light
- Ortho chromatic emulsion—sensitive to *GREEN* light
- Pan chromatic emulsion—sensitive to *RED* light.

Sharpness and speed of the film depends on size of the silver halide grains. Faster films have larger grain size and required less radiation on contrary produce less contrast.

Kodak has introduces new films (T-mat) with tabular shaped silver halide grains are oriented with their flat faces to the radiation providing a larger surface resulting in increased speed without loss of sharpness.

INTENSIFYING SCREENS

Intensifying screens are image receptor system, used in combination with X-ray film for all extraoral radiographic procedure such as panoramic, cephalometric and skull radiography.

Types: Two types of intensifying screens are available depending on emitting light:

1. Blue emitting visible light.
2. Green emitting visible light.

Mechanism

Intensifying screens contains various inorganic salts or phosphors would fluorescence (emit visible light) when exposed to an X-ray beam. The intensity of this fluorescence is directly proportional to intensity of the X-ray beam, which strike the phosphors crystal.

Each X-ray photon convert into multiple visible light which strikes the X-ray film thus reducing amount of radiation required to expose film, but resulting in loss of fine detail on image because of dispersion of visible lights from phosphor crystals **(Fig. 8.1A)**.

Composition

Intensifying screen contains **(Fig. 8.1B)**:

- Base
- Reflecting layer
- Phosphor layer
- Protective coat.

Base: It is made up of *polyester plastic* with 0.25 mm thickness which provides mechanical support for the intensifying screen.

Reflecting layer: It is made up of *Titanium Dioxide,* coated on the base material and lies below the phosphor layer. The main function is to reflect any visible light emitted from the phosphor layer back to the X-ray film. Devoid this layer in some intensifying screens to get a sharpness of the image because this layer produce divergence of the visible light reflected back to film causing unsharpened of the image.

Phosphor layer: Phosphor layer composed of light sensitive phosphor crystals suspended in a plastic material. When the phosphors are struck by X-ray photons they emit visible light that exposes the X-ray film.

Most common phosphor used in dentistry and medicines are *calcium tungstate,* which emit blue visible light. In recent years rare

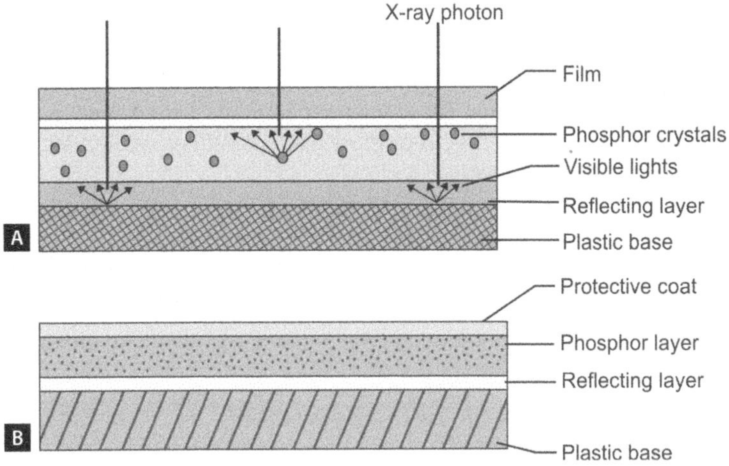

Figs 8.1A and B: (A) Mechanism of action of intensifying screen; (B) Cross-section of intensifying screen contains base, reflecting layer, phosphor and protective layer

earth elements such as *Terbium activated, Gadolinium oxysulfide* and *Thulium-activated lanthanum oxybromide* have been used. These are generally more advantageous in that they are four times more efficient than calcium tungstate in converting X-ray photons into visible light and they are in green emission spectrum. Large phosphor crystal size increases the speed of the intensifying screen there by reducing the exposure time but the image clarity will be reduced and vice versa.

Protective coat: It is made up of plastic about 8 mm thickness placed over the phosphor layer to provide protection for the phosphor layer.

GRIDS

A grid is an alternative strip of radiopaque and radiolucent material is placed between the object and the film to improve the quality of the image by removal of scattered radiation that causes fog and reduces film contrast.

Composition

It is composed of alternate strips of radiopaque that are lead and radiolucent often plastic material.

Functions

When X-ray photons hits the object (patient's head) secondary photons generated in the object by Compton effect of radiation and they are scattered towards the film. These scattered photons are deviated in their direction of travel from that of primary beam would cause film fog and reducing the film contrast.

Grids are placed between the object and the films absorbs all scattered radiation that are deviated from the primary X-ray beam by radiopaque material that consists of lead and allow only primary beam through the radiolucent material of plastic into the film thereby reducing film fog and contrast.

Types of Grids

Two types of grids:

1. *Stationary grids:*
   - Parallel grid
   - Focused grid
2. *Moving grids:*
   - Bucky grid

Stationary Grids

- *Parallel grid:* In parallel grid secondary radiation originated in the object are absorbed by the parallely placed radiopaque lead strips. Radiolucent plastic strips allow primary beam and few secondary beams, which are in the direction of primary beam towards the film **(Fig. 8.2)**.

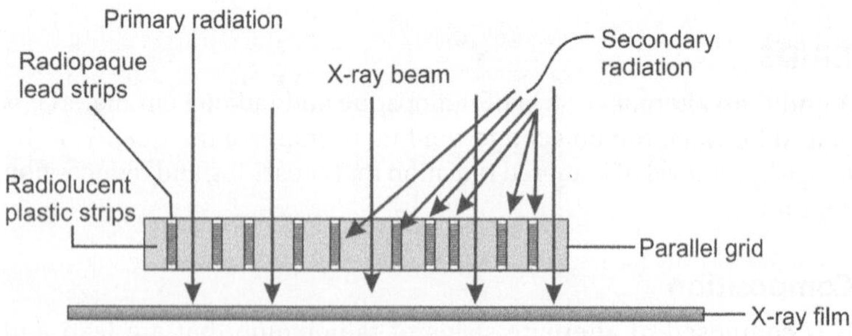

Fig. 8.2: Parallel-placed radiolucent and radiopaque strips allow primary beam and stops secondary radiation which travels in different direction of primary radiations

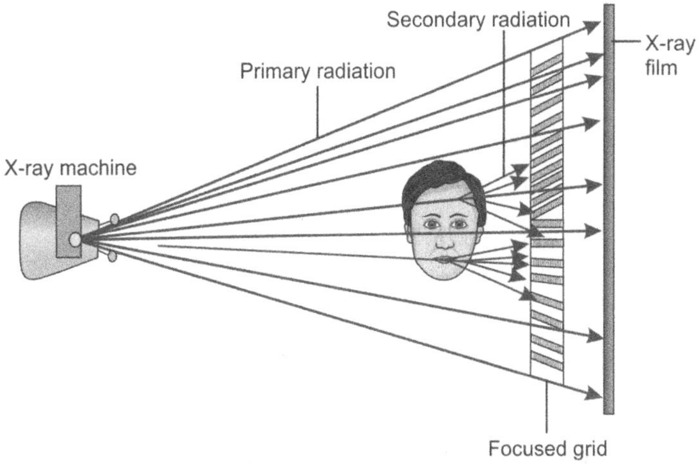

Fig. 8.3: Focused grid shows strips of radiopaque directs towards the common point where all the information carrying rays are passed through it

- *Focused grid:* It is used most frequently. In focused grid, strips of radiopaque material are directed towards the common point. Their direction is coincides with the direction of the paths of the diverging secondary photons, thereby eliminate the absorption of more secondary radiation than parallel grid **(Fig. 8.3)**.

Moving Grids

- *Bucky grid:* These are the moving grids which move mechanically in the direction of 90° to the grid lines during exposure. This movement of grid cause blurring out the radiolucent lines of image produced in case of other types of grids and result in uniform exposure.

Presence of radiopaque and radiolucent material results in the images of white and dark lines over the films. To reduce this, grids are manufactured with variable number of line pairs of radiopaque and lucent strips per inch. Usually, grids with 80 lines pair/inch do not show the grid lines over the image.

Grid ratio: Ratio of the thickness of the grid to the width of the radiolucent is known as the grid ratio.

Grid ratio = Width of the radiolucent/thickness of the grid.

The higher the grid ratio the more effectively remove the scattered radiation from the X-ray beam. Normal grid ratio is 8–10 are usually preferred.

EXTRAORAL RADIOGRAPHIC TECHNIQUES

Extraoral radiography includes all views made of the orofacial region with films positioned extraorally such as:

Skull Projections

- Posteroanterior projections (PA view)
- Lateral skull projections (lateral cephalometric projections)
- Water's projections (PNS view or occipitomental projections)
- Reverse Towne's projections
- Submentovertex projections.

Mandibular Oblique Lateral Projections

(a) Mandibular body projections and (b) Mandibular ramus projections

Temporomandibular Projections

(a) Transpharyngeal, (b) Transcranial and (c) Transorbital.

Tomography (Discussed in Chapter 10)

- Conventional tomography
- Computed tomography
- Three-dimensional computed tomography (CBCT)
- Spiral computed tomography
- Emission computed tomography (PET and SPECT scan)

Paranasal Sinus Projections

- Frontal sinus
- Ethmoidal
- Sphenoidal
- Maxillary sinus

To achieve the best images with the lowest exposures, it is important to make all extraoral radiographic projections with the appropriate combination of film and intensifying screen. Medium or high-speed rare earth screen film combination provides best image detail with less radiation exposure to patient. For lateral oblique views of mandible 5 × 7″ film and cassette are sufficient. A skull film requires at least 8 × 10″ film and cassette.

The positioning of patient for the different skull projections is facilitated by the use of two anatomical land marks, *Canthomeatal line* (A line joins outer canthus of the eye to external auditory meatus of the ear) and other one is *Frankfort line* (A line joining from external auditory meatus to infraorbital rim **(Fig. 8.4)**.

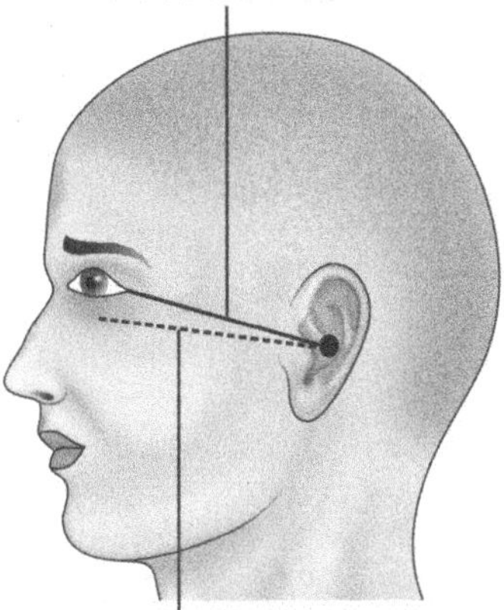

Fig. 8.4: Canthomeatal and Frankfort anatomical landmark lines used to position the patient for the skull radiographs

SKULL PROJECTIONS

Posteroanterior Projections

It is so named because the X-ray beam passes in a posterior to anterior direction through the skull **(Fig. 8.5)**.

Indications

- Examine the skull for disease, trauma or developmental abnormalities.
- Provides a good record for detecting progressive changes in the mediolateral dimensions of the skull including asymmetric growth.
- Good visualization of facial structures including frontal, ethmoidal sinus, nasal fossa and orbits.

Head Position

For the straight PA projection the head is centered in front of the cassette with the canthomeatal line parallel to the floor.

Beam Alignment

The central ray directed through the center of the head and perpendicular to the cassette **(Fig. 8.6)**.

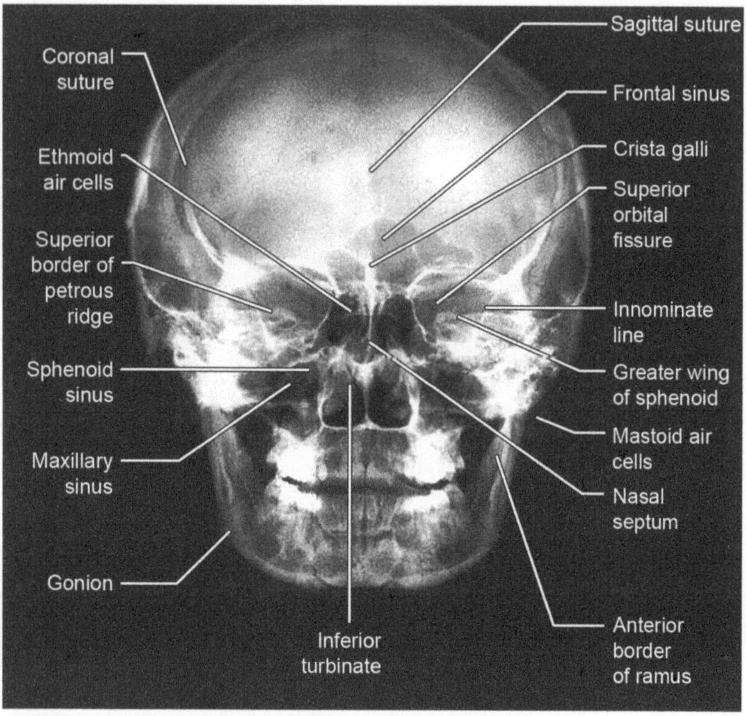

Fig. 8.5: Posteroanterior radiograph

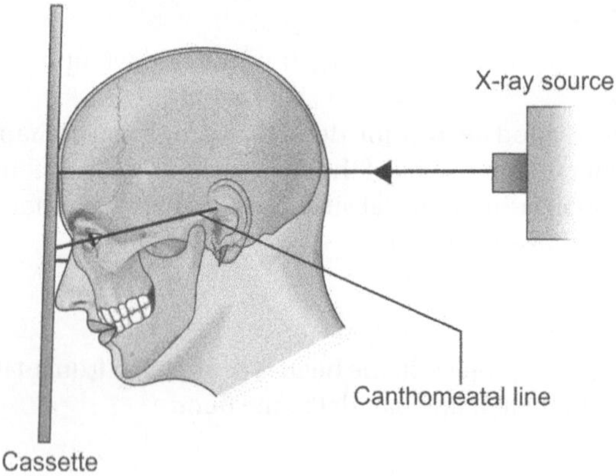

Fig. 8.6: Patient position and projection of X-ray beam

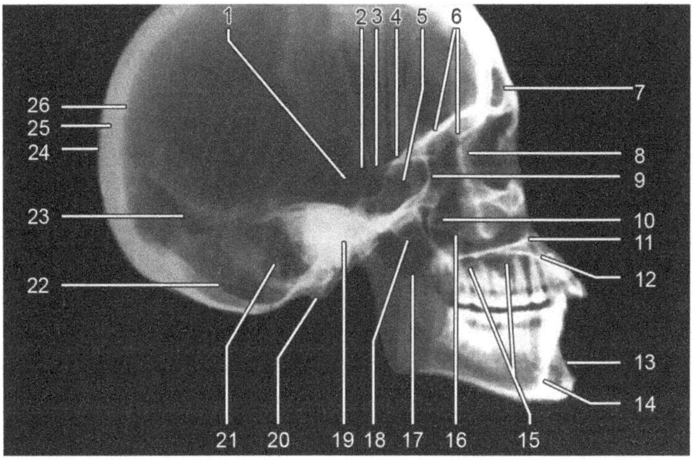

1. Posterior clinoid process
2. Sella turcica (Pituitary fossa)
3. Anterior clinoid process
4. Floor of anterior cranial fossa in the midline
5. Sphenoid sinus
6. Orbital plates of frontal bone
7. Frontal sinus
8. Lateral border of orbit
9. Greater wing of the sphenoid bone
10. Pterygomaxillary fissure
11. Hard palate
12. Roof of palate (midline)
13. Buccal cortical plate of anterior portion of mandible
14. Lingual cortical plate
15. Floor of maxillary sinus
16. Zygoma
17. Sigmoid notch (mandibular notch)
18. Lateral pterygoid plate
19. Petrous portion of temporal bone
20. Mastoid process of temporal bone
21. Mastoid air cells
22. Occipital bone
23. Lambdoid suture
24. Outer cortex of bone
25. Diploe
26. Inner cortex of bone

Fig. 8.7: Lateral cephalometric radiograph

For PA cephalometric projection the head is slightly upward so that canthomeatal line 10° above the horizontal plane, i.e. Frankfort plane is perpendicular to the film or parallel to the floor.

Lateral Skull Projections (Lateral Cephalometric Projection) (Fig. 8.7)

Indications

- Survey the skull and facial bones for evidence of trauma disease or developmental abnormality.

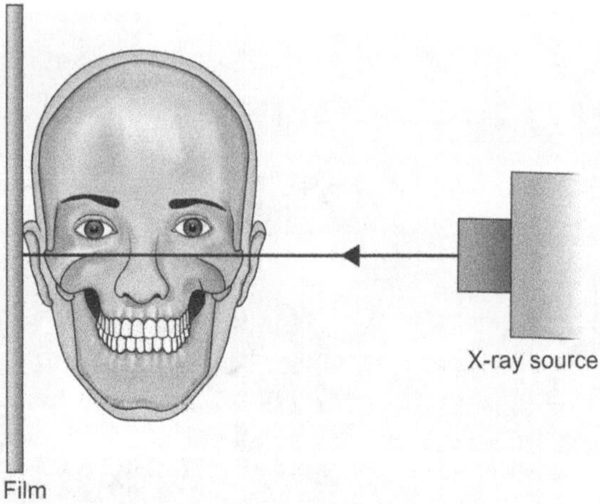

Fig. 8.8: Patient and the cassette positioning for lateral cephalometry

- Reveals the nasopharyngeal soft tissue, paranasal sinus and hard palate.
- Mainly used in orthodontics to assess facial growth.
- Used in oral surgery and prosthodontics to establish pretreatment and post treatment records.

Head Position

Head should be positioned with the left side of the face near the cassette. A wedge filter is placed over the anterior side of the beam at the tube head. The filter absorbs some of the radiation striking the facial soft tissue thereby reducing the intensity of radiation and obtaining soft tissue outline of the patients face on the radiograph.

The central ray is directed towards the external auditory meatus and perpendicular to the plane of the film **(Fig. 8.8)**.

Water's Projections or PNS View (Fig. 8.9)

Indications

- To evaluate the disease in paranasal sinus especially in case of maxillary sinusitis.
- To examine the Le Fort II and III fractures
- To examine the fracture of coronoid process of the mandible.

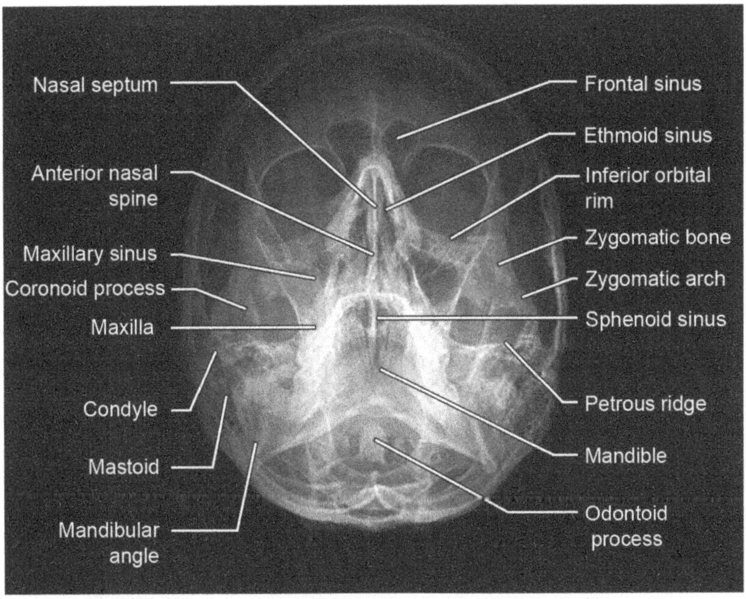

Fig. 8.9: Paranasal sinus radiograph

Head Position

Head should be oriented with sagittal plane perpendicular to the plane of the film. The chin is raised high to elevate the canthomeatal line 37° above the horizontal plane and ask the patient to open the mouth so that image of the sphenoid sinus will project on to the palate.

The central ray directed to the film at the level of the maxillary sinus **(Fig. 8.10)**.

Reverse Towne's Projections (Fig. 8.11)

Indications

- To examine the condylar neck fracture.
- To reveal the posterolateral wall of the maxillary antrum.

Head Position

Head should be centered and downward in front of the cassette with the canthomeatal line is 25°–30° downward to the horizontal plane, and mouth should be kept open as wide as possible. The central beam directed toward the film in the sagittal plane through the occipital bone **(Fig. 8.12)**.

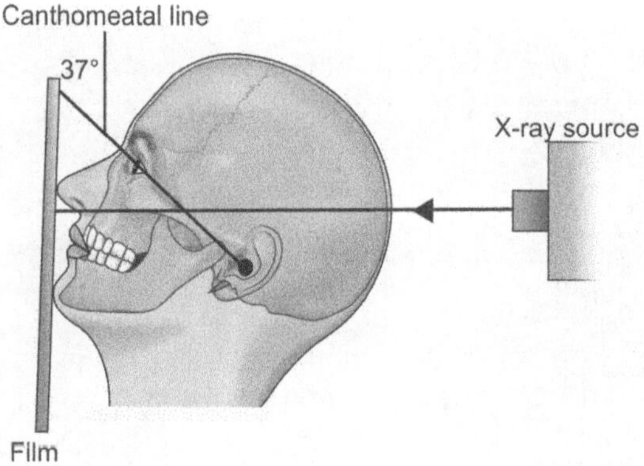

Fig. 8.10: Positioning of patient head with respect to cassette for PNS projections

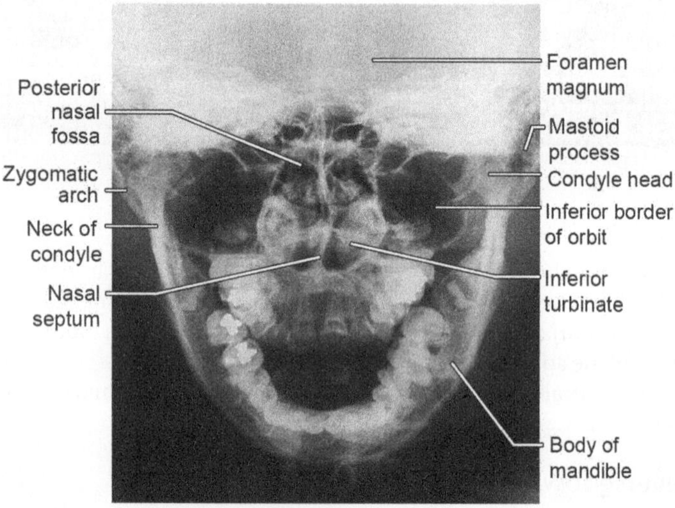

Fig. 8.11: Reverse Towne's view

Submentovertex Projections

Indications

- To demonstrate the base of the skull **(Fig. 8.13)**.
- To examine the position and orientation of the condyle and sphenoid sinus.
- To reveal the # zygomatic arch of the maxilla **(Fig. 8.14)**.
- To assess the medial and lateral pterygoid plates.

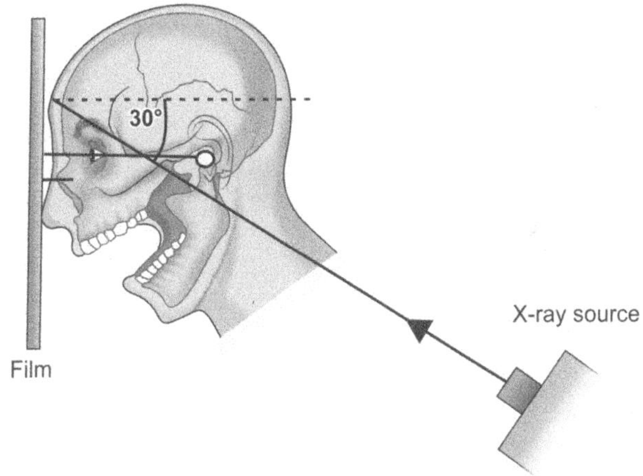

Fig. 8.12: Patient head should be 25°–30° downward to the horizontal plane for reverse Towne's projections

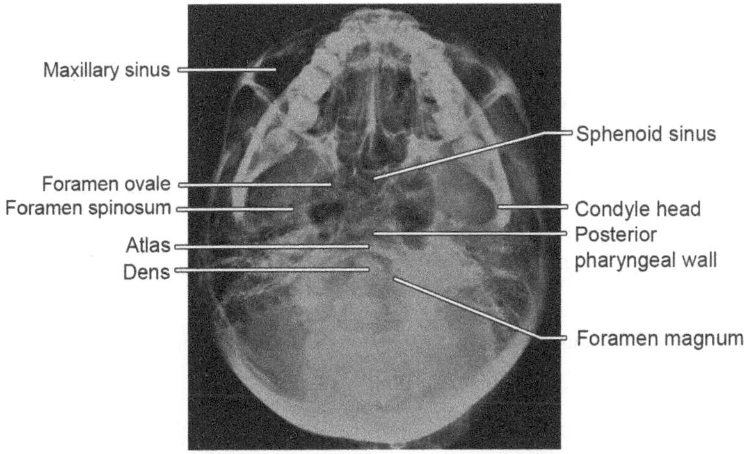

Fig. 8.13: Submentovertex radiograph showing base of the skull

Head Position

The patient's head and neck should be hyperextended backward with the vertex of the skull on the center of the cassette. The canthomeatal line should be 10° past vertical so that FH plane is vertical and parallel to the film.

The central ray is directed from below the mandible **(Fig. 8.15)**.

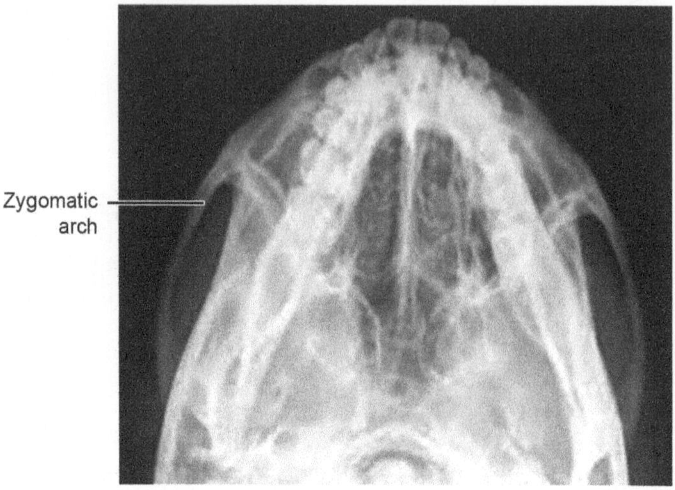

Fig. 8.14: Submentovertex radiograph showing zygomatic arch of the maxilla

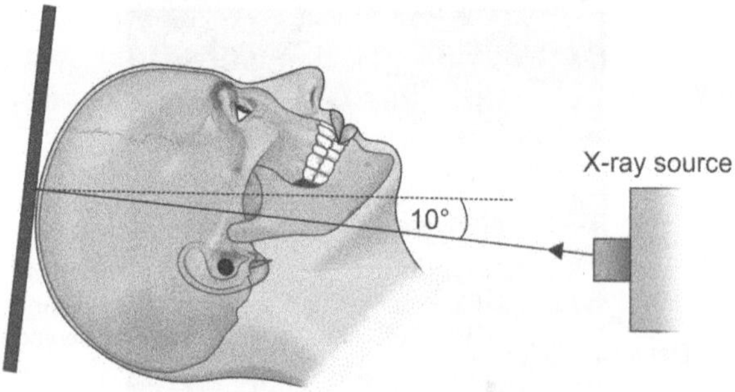

Fig. 8.15: Adjust the patient's head such that canthomeatal line is 10° past vertical plane for submentovertex projection

When specifically desired to view the zygomatic arches, the exposure time should be reduced to one-third of that used to view the base of the skull.

MANDIBULAR OBLIQUE LATERAL PROJECTIONS

These projections commonly used to examine the mandible when the patient is under trismus and cannot be able to allow taking intraoral radiographs. There are two projections:

1. Mandibular body projection
2. Mandibular ramus projection

Mandibular Body Projection (Fig. 8.16)

Indications

- To demonstrate any pathology in premolar and molar region impossible to achieve in intraoral radiographs.
- To view the broader coverage of periapical area.
- Patient is under trismus.

Film Placement

Cassette is placed against the patient's cheek and centered over the 1st molar. Its lower surface parallel with the inferior border of the mandible and extending 2 cm below it. The patient can hold the cassette in place. The head is tilted toward the side being examined and the mandible is protruded to avoid the vertebral superimposition.

The central ray directed 2 cm below the angle of the mandible in the 1st molar region directed anteriorly.

Mandibular Ramus Projection (Fig. 8.16)

Indications

- To view the pathology in ramus region.
- To demonstrate pathology in the 3rd molar area of maxilla and mandible.
- In case of trismus.

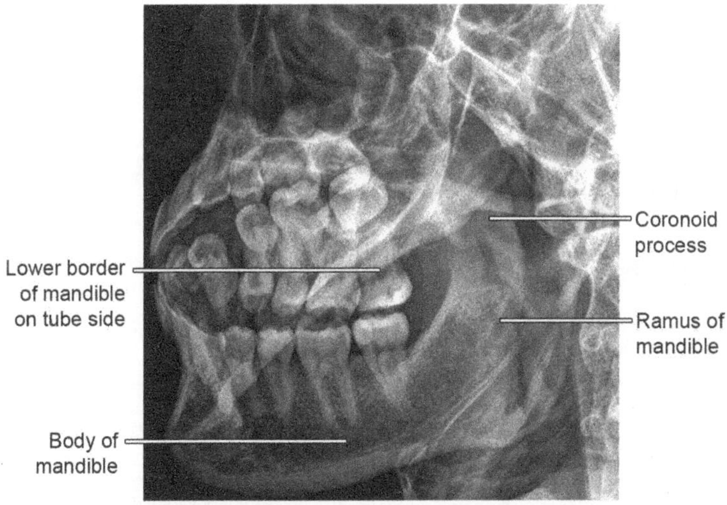

Fig. 8.16: Mandibular oblique lateral projections showing body and ramus of the mandible

Film Placement

The cassette is placed over the ramus to include the condyle. The lower border of the cassette is parallel with the inferior border of the mandible and should extend 2 cm below the border.

Head Position

Head is tilted toward the side of the mandible being examined and mandible is protruded to prevent the cervical spine being superimposed over the ramus.

The central ray directed posteriorly toward the center of the ramus on the side of interest from a point 2 cm below the inferior border of the 1st molar region of the mandible on the tube side **(Fig. 8.16)**.

TEMPOROMANDIBULAR JOINT PROJECTIONS

Temporomandibular joint (TMJ) is a complex structure. Radiographic projections of the TMJ is very difficult because of its anatomical locations. Hence different radiographic projections are selected to view the all the surface of the joint. The type of imaging technique selected depends on the specific clinical problem, whether imaging of hard or soft tissues of TMJ is desired **(Table 8.1)**.

Table 8.1: Summary of the different parts of the TMJ by the main radiographic projections

Radiographic investigations	*Area of joint shown*
Transcranial	**Lateral aspect of:** • Glenoid fossa • Joint space • Articular eminence • Condylar head
Transpharyngeal	**Lateral view of:** • Condylar head and neck • Articular surface
Transorbital	**Anterior view of:** • Condylar head and neck • Articular surface
Dental panoramic tomography	**Lateral view of:** Both condylar heads
Reverse Towne's	**Posterior view of:** Both condylar heads and necks
Tomography	**All aspects of:** • Glenoid fossa • Articular eminence joint space • Condylar head

TMJ hard tissue imaging to evaluate the osseous contours, condyle and fossa.

Hard tissue TMJ projections:
- Panoramic radiograph
- Transcranial projection
- Transpharyngeal (Parma) projection
- Transorbital projection
- Submentovertex projection
- Computed tomography

Soft tissue TMJ imaging is indicated when information about disk position, morphology and surrounding tissue.

Soft tissues of the joint can be imaged by:
- Arthrography
- MRI

Transcranial Projection

Indications (**Figs 8.17A and B**)

- To view the changes in the lateral aspects of the condylar head and articular fossa in arthritis.
- To evaluate the condylar position in the mandibular fossa.
- To view the fracture of condylar head.

Procedure

Cassette is positioned against the facial skin surface on the side of interest, parallel to the sagittal plane. X-ray beam projects from behind

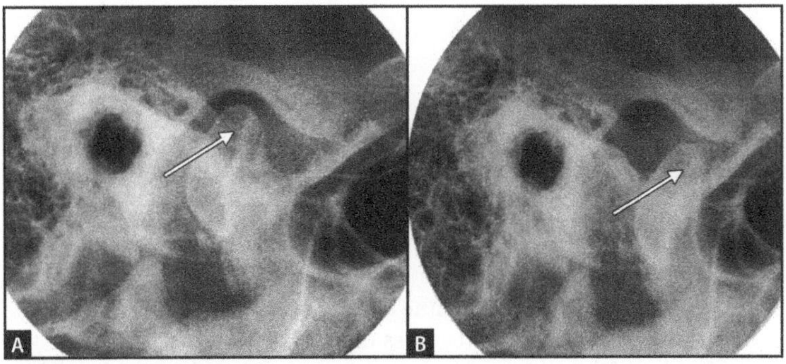

Figs 8.17A and B: Transcranial TMJ projection shows lateral aspect of condyle in (A) Closed position; (B) Open position of condyle

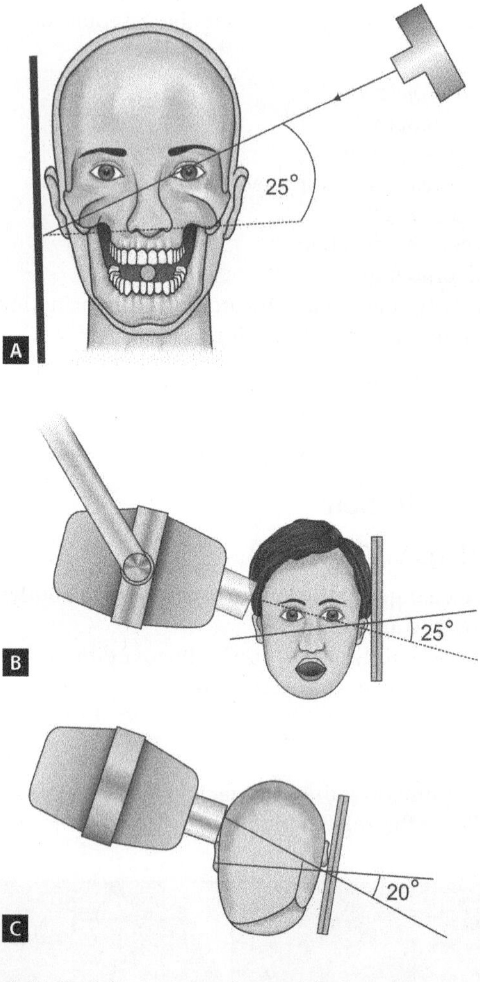

Figs 8.18A to C: (A) Skull diagram showing positioning of X-ray cone and the film. (B) X-ray beam project from behind the head at an angulation of 25° downward to the horizontal plane. (C) Central beam pass across the cranium at 20° anterior to the horizontal plane

the head in such a way that central ray should pass 25° downward and 20° anterior to the horizontal plane and is centered on the TMJ.

Central beam is projected across the cranium passes just above the petrous ridge of the temporal bone on the film side **(Figs 8.18A to C)**.

Transpharyngeal or Parma or McQueen or Infracranial Projection

Indications (Fig. 8.19)

- To view the fracture of the condyle and neck.
- To detect gross alterations in condyle.
- To evaluate pathology involved in the condyle and mandibular ramus region.

Procedure

Cassette is positioned on the side of interest. Central ray projects 5–10° upward and 10° posterior to the horizontal plane and centered over the TMJ of interesting side.

Central beam projects through the sigmoid notch (Window between the condyle and coronoid process). Before exposure, ask the patient open the mouth wide so that:

- Condyle moves out of osseous structure into soft tissue region so that better view the condyle is possible.
- It enlarges the window between the mandibular notch and zygomatic process through which central X-ray beam must pass **(Figs 8.20A to C)**.

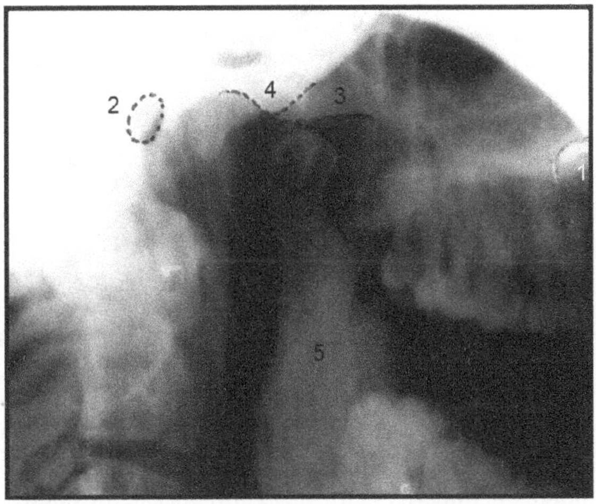

Fig. 8.19: Transpharyngeal radiograph showing lateral aspect of condyle
1. Head of condyle; 2. External auditory meatus; 3. Articular eminence; 4. Glenoid fossa; 5. Neck of the condyle

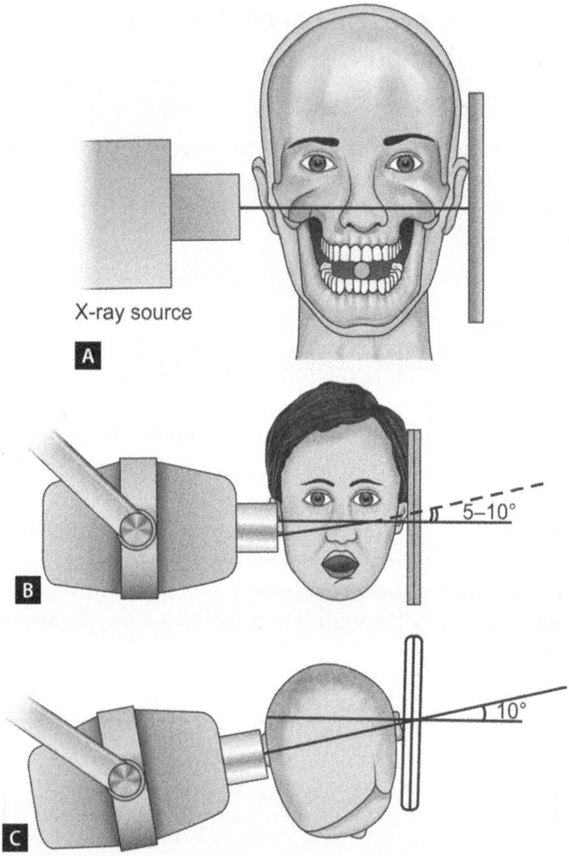

Figs 8.20A to C: (A) Diagram of skull shows patient and film position; (B) Central beam projects through sigmoid notch and pass at 5–10° upward to the horizontal plane; (C) Beam pass at 10° backwards to the horizontal plane

Transorbital or Transmaxillary or Zimmer Projections

Indications **(Fig. 8.21)**

- To visualization of entire mediolateral articulating surfaces of the condyle and articular eminence.
- To evaluate the integrity of the head and neck of the condyle.

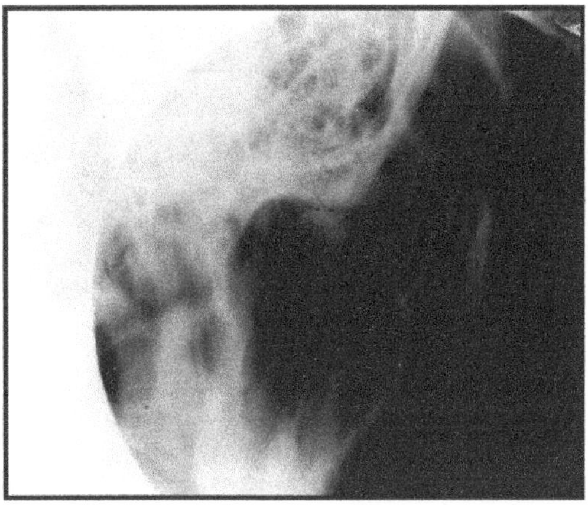

Fig. 8.21: Transorbital radiograph showing condyle and articulating surface

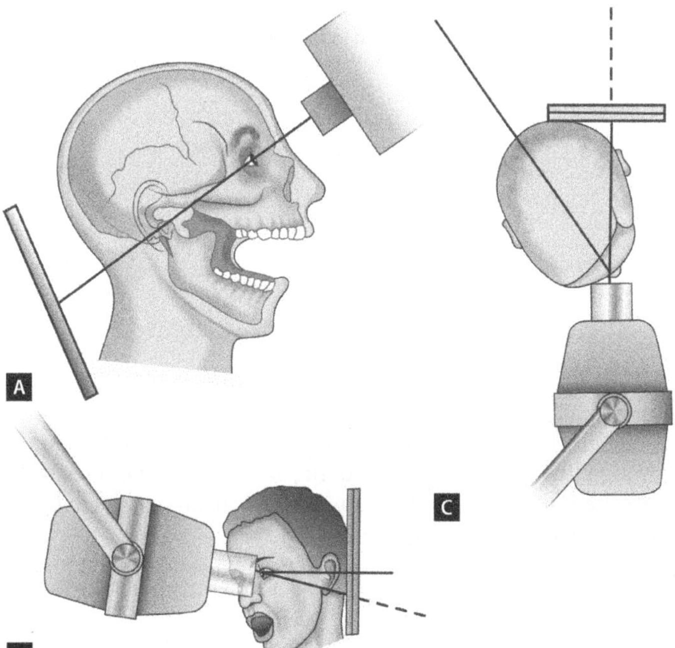

Figs 8.22A to C: (A) Skull diagram showing X-ray cone and the film placement; (B) X-ray beam is projected 10° downward; (C) X-ray beam pass laterally 30° through ipsilateral orbit

Table 8.2: Summary of the different radiographic investigations that can be used for the various paranasal air sinuses

Air sinus	*Radiographic investigations*
Frontal	• Occipitomental (PNS) • PA view of skull • True lateral skull • Tomography • Computed tomography (CT) • Magnetic resonance imaging (MRI)
Sphenoidal	• Occipitomental (with the patient's mouth open) • True lateral skull • Submentovertex (SMV) • Tomography • Computed tomography (CT) • Magnetic resonance imaging (MRI)
Ethmoidal	• Occipitomental • True lateral skull • PA view of skull • Tomography • Computed tomography (CT) • Magnetic resonance imaging (MRI)
Maxillary	• Occipitomental (PNS view) • PA view of skull • Orthopantomography (OPG) • True lateral skull • Submentovertex • Computed tomography (CT) • Magnetic resonance imaging (MRI)

Procedure

- Patient position should be such that canthomeatal line should be horizontal.
- X-ray tube is placed in front of the patient and directs the central ray through the ipsilateral orbit and through the TMJ of interest side.
- Cassette is positioned behind the patient's head so that central ray is projected to its center.
- Ask the patient to open the mouth as wide as possible to move the condyle out of the articular fossa **(Figs 8.22A to C)**.

Paranasal Sinus Projections

The different radiographic investigations used for various paranasal air sinuses are summarized in **Table 8.2**.

CHAPTER 9

Panoramic Radiography

INTRODUCTION

Panoramic radiography or pantomography or rotational radiography is a radiographic procedure that produces a single image of the facial structures, including both maxillary and mandibular arches and their supporting structures **(Figs 9.1 and 9.2)**.

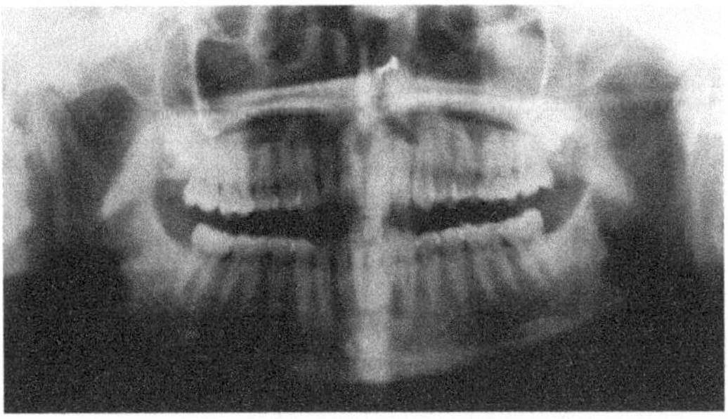

Fig. 9.1: Panoramic radiograph

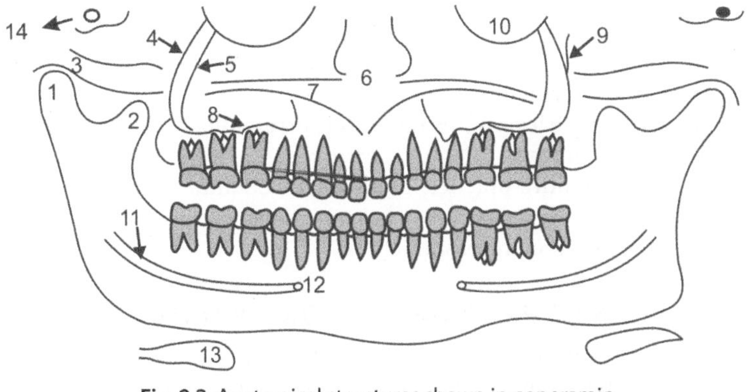

Fig. 9.2: Anatomical structures shown in panoramic

1. Mandibular condyle; 2. Coronoid process; 3. Zygomatic arch; 4. Posterior wall of maxillary sinus; 5. Posterior wall of zygomatic process; 6. Nasal septum; 7. Hard palate; 8. Inferior border of maxillary sinus; 9. Anterior border of pterygoid plates; 10: Orbit; 11. Mandibular canal; 12. Mental foramen; 13. Hyoid bone; 14. Middle cranial fossa.

Advantages

- Broad anatomic region imaged
- Low patient radiation dose.
- Convenience to the patient and the operator.
- Performed on patient with trismus.
- Used as a visual aid in case presentation and patient education.

Disadvantages

- Image does not resolve fine anatomic detail that may be seen on intraoral periapical radiographs.
- Magnification, geometric distortion and overlapped images of tooth, especially in the premolar region.
- Objects lie outside the focal trough being distorted or blurred on the resultant radiograph.
- The cost of the machine is 2–4 times more than intraoral X-ray machine.

In spite of these disadvantages, panoramic radiographs can be very useful in many diagnostic examinations.

Indications

- To evaluate the trauma to the Jaws especially mandible.
- To evaluate the third molar and surrounding region.
- To examine the extensive pathology of Jaws.
- To evaluate the tooth development specially in mixed dentition analysis
- To evaluate developmental anomalies of tooth like anodontia **(Fig. 9.3)**, etc.
- Useful aid in orthodontic treatment.
- To measure the level of the bone and surrounding structures in case of implant surgery.
- In prosthodontics practice, measure the edentulous gap to fix the bridge.
- For general screening examination.

PRINCIPLES OF PANORAMIC RADIOGRAPHY

It was first described by *Numata* (1933) and *Paatero* (1948). The principles of panoramic radiograph can be understood by considering the following illustrations.

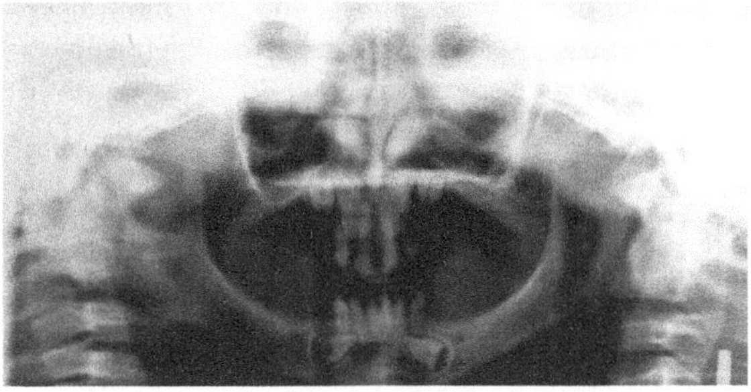

Fig. 9.3: Panoramic radiograph shows partial anodontia

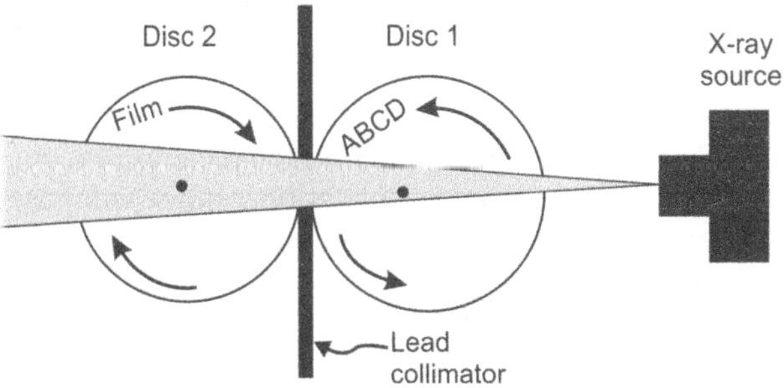

Fig. 9.4: Illustration 1: Movement of film and objects about two fixed centers of rotation

1st Illustration

Consider two adjacent discs rotating at the same speed in opposite direction (disc 1 rotating anticlockwise and disc 2 clockwise). X-ray beam is directed through their centers of rotation. Lead collimator in the shape of a slit located at the X-ray source and film limit the central ray to a narrow slit beam. The object ABCD on disc 1 rotate past the slit, and their images are recorded on the film, i.e. disc 2. The objects will be sharply revealed on the film because they are moving past the slit at the same rate as the film **(Fig. 9.4)**.

2nd Illustration

In 2nd illustration X-ray source is rotated so that the central ray constantly passed through the center of rotation of disc 1 and simultaneously both disc 2 and the collimator rotate about the center of disc 1.Optimum image definition obtained when the speed of the film (disc 2) equal to the speed of the X-ray source which sweeps through the objects of ABCD on disc 1. Here both X-ray source and the film (disc 2) moved at a same speed in opposite direction at one fixed center of rotation **(Fig. 9.5)**.

3rd Illustration

3rd illustration shows that disc 1 may be replaced with a patient. During the exposure cycle the machine will automatically shift to other rotation centers. The movement of the film is equal to the speed of the X-ray source that sweeps through the dental structure of the patient near the film. Structures on the other side of the patient (near the X-ray tube) are distorted and magnified that they are not visible (blurred off) because they are in out of the focus area. Thus only structures near the film will be usefully imaged on the resultant radiograph **(Fig. 9.6)**.

Focal trough: Focal trough is a three-dimensional curved zone or image layer in which structures are well-defined on panoramic radiographs.

The image seen on a panoramic radiograph is composed largely of the anatomic structures located within the focal trough. Objects in front or behind the focal trough are appears blurred or distorted on the resultant radiograph so that they are not recognizable.

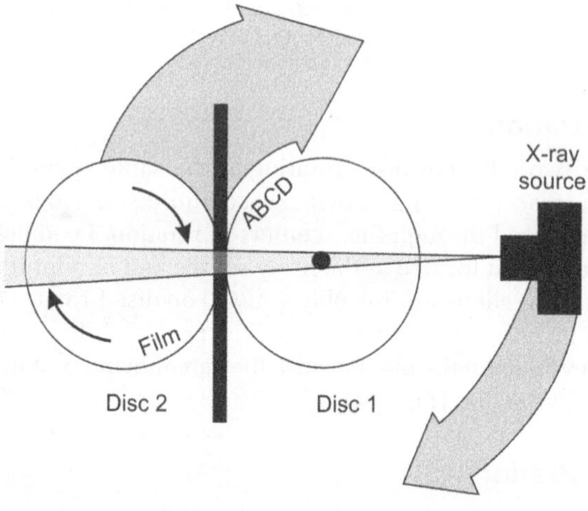

Fig. 9.5: Illustration 2: movement of film and X-ray source at one fixed center of rotation

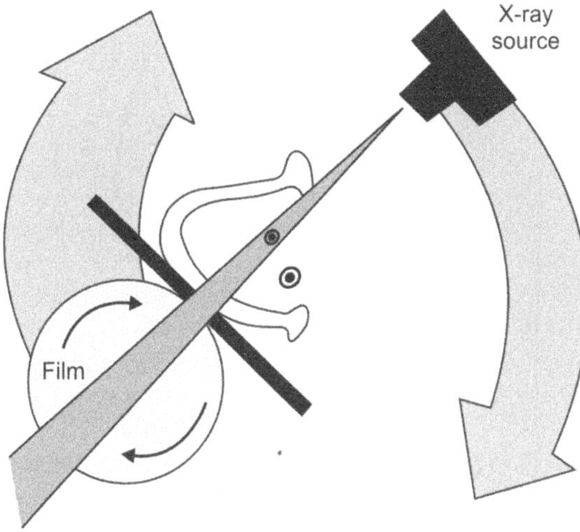

Fig. 9.6: Illustration 3: During movement of film and X-ray source around the patient, machine automatically shift to other center of rotation

The shape of the focal trough varies with the brand of panoramic machine used. **Figure 9.7** shows the general shape of the focal trough used in panoramic machines.

If the object or patient jaw positioned anterior to the focal trough will cause decreased width of the images of teeth (overlapping of tooth). Image appeared increased in width (magnification of tooth) when the object lies posterior or behind the focal trough.

PATIENT POSITIONING AND HEAD ALIGNMENT

Patient positioned correctly in the panoramic machine so that jaws and teeth are with in the focal trough.

- Removal of glasses, metallic items such as earrings, necklace, hairpins, nose rings, hearing aids and dental appliances.
- Explain the patient to remain still during the exposure.
- Instruct the patient to look forward and not follow the X-ray tube head.
- Should stand erect or straight with back straight.
- Patient head should be tilted slightly downward so that occlusal plane should be parallel to the floor.
- Align the mid-sagittal plane of the patient's head with the vertical central line of chin rest.

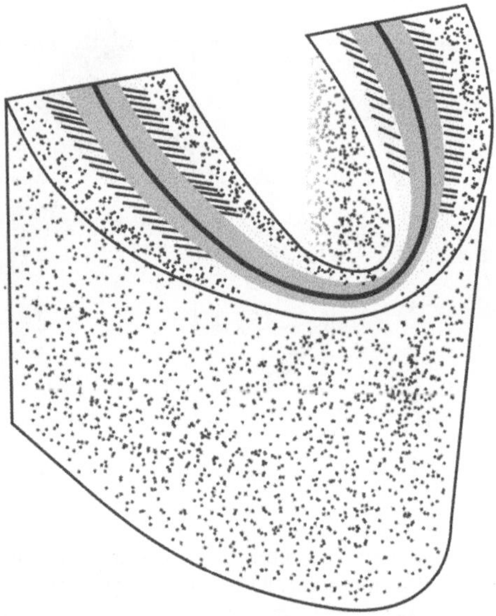

Fig. 9.7: Focal trough showing anatomical structures at the center of the trough (dark zone) appears clearer than adjacent structures on the radiograph

- Ask the patient to bite over the bite block with both maxillary and mandibular incisors.
- Ask patient to close the lips and place the tongue against the hard palate.

FAULTS IN PATIENT POSITIONING (TABLE 9.1)

- If the chin and the occlusal plane upward resulting in widening of teeth and shadow of hard palate superimpose over the apices of maxillary teeth.
- If the patient's chin is tipped downward, the tooth becomes severely overlapped. Symphyseal region of the mandible may be cutoff the film and both condyles may be projected top of the film. A general guide line for chin positioning is to place the patient in such way that FH plane is parallel to the floor.
- Proper patient positioning also requires positioning the patient's back and spine in an erect position with the neck extended. Slumping causes a large opaque artifact of cervical spine superimpose over the symphyseal region of the mandible.

Table 9.1: Summary of errors and correction of patient's position during panoramic radiographic procedures

Positioning errors	*Resultant image*	*Correction*
1. Chin and occlusal plane kept upward	Widening of teeth and shadow of hard palate superimpose over the apices of maxillary teeth	Make the patient's head in such a way that FH plane parallel to the floor
2. Chin and occlusal plane kept downward	Narrow and overlapped of teeth. Symphyseal region of image may cut-off and both condyles projected at top	Make the patient's head in such a way that FH plane parallel to the floor
3. Patient's is in slumping position	Large opaque artifact of cervical spine superimpose over the symphyseal region	Patient's back and spine should be erect and neck extended
4. If the incisors are positioned infront of the bite block notch (anterior to the focal trough)	Decreased in width of the teeth image (vertical magnification)	Incisors positioned exactly into the bite block notch, so that dental arch in focal trough
5. Incisors positioned back of the bite block notch (posterior to the focal trough)	Increased width of the teeth image (horizontal magnification)	Incisors positioned exactly into the bite block notch, so that dental arch in focal trough
6. Failure to position the patient in midsagittal plane	Unequal horizontal magnification either left or right side	Position the patient into the midsagittal plane
7. Accidental movement of patient's head during exposure	Blurring or magnified image	Patient's head should be positioned within the head rest and chin on the chin rest
8. Failure to position the tongue against the palate	Radiolucent line run across the angle of the mandible mimics the fracture	Instruct the patient to place the tongue against the palate so that no airway space between soft palate and dorsum of the tongue
9. Failure to remove the metal earrings, chain, hair pin and nose ring	Ghost image formed that obscure the resultant image details	Instruct the patient to remove all head and neck metal ornaments

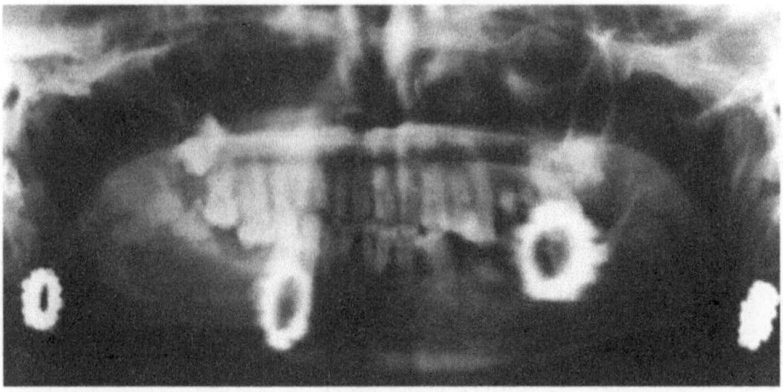

Fig. 9.8: Ghost image appeared on panoramic radiography

- Proper patient positioning requires placing the patient so that dental arch is located in the center of the focal trough. This can be accomplished by place the maxilla and mandibular incisors in a bite block.

  If the incisors are positioned anterior to the bite block (anterior to the focal trough) the resultant image decreased in width (vertical magnification).

  If the incisors are posterior to the bite block results in increased width of the image (horizontal magnification).
- Failure to position the patient in midsagittal plane results in unequal horizontal magnification either left or right side.
- Patient tongue positioned against the palate. Failure to do this result in an radiolucent line run across the angle of the mandible mimic fracture at angle of the mandible obtained by the air space between the dorsum of the tongue and the soft palate.

Ghost image: Radiopaque shadows that superimpose over normal anatomic structures are called Ghost image, which are artifact.

They result when the X-ray beam is projected through a dense object, such as earrings, spinal column, mandible and hard palate. The opaque shadow of the object (ghost) is projected on to the opposite side of the radiograph, which obscures the normal radiographic interpretation **(Fig. 9.8)**.

CHAPTER

10 Specialized Radiographic Techniques

Specialized radiographic techniques are not used routinely, occasionally used to aid in diagnosis of certain conditions in the oral cavity.

TYPES

- *Tomography:*
  - Conventional tomography
  - Computed tomography (CT scan)
  - Emission tomography (PET or SPECT scan)
- Stereoscopy
- Scanography
- *Digital imaging:*
  - Direct
  - Indirect
- Magnetic resonance imaging (MRI)
- Nuclear medicine or scintigraphy
- Ultrasonography
- Electronic thermography.

CONVENTIONAL TOMOGRAPHY

Conventional or body section radiography is a radiographic technique designed to image more clearly, when objects lying within a plane of interest. This is accomplished by blurring the images of structures lying superficial and deep to the plane of interest through the process of motion unsharpness **(Fig. 10.1)**.

The objective of tomography is to blur the images of structures not located in the focal plane. Blurring is greater under the following conditions.

- The farther the object lies from the focal plane and the greater the distance between object and the film.
- Long axis of the objects is located superficial or deep to the focal plane lie parallel with the path of the X-ray tube and film movement.

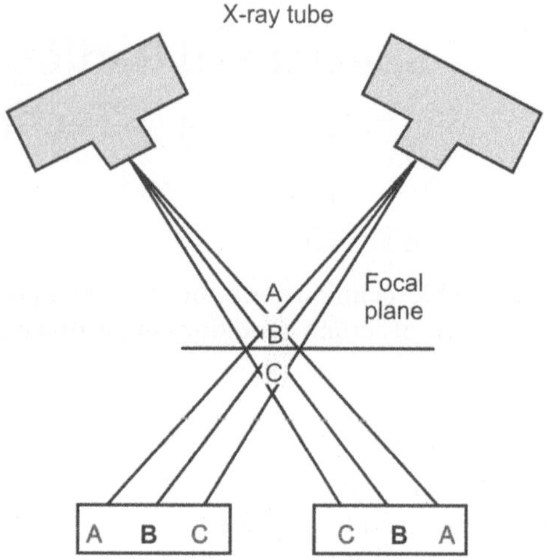

Fig. 10.1: Tomographic techniques. X-ray tube moves from left to right and film moves in opposite direction. In the figure, point B lies at the focal plane appears sharp and other points A, C out of focal plane appears blurred

Tomographic movements: There are different types of tomographic motion. The thickness of tissue in the focal plane is called the tomographic layer. The relationship between the tomographic angle and the thickness of object is described as, *Greater the tomographic angle, the thinner the object thickness and vice versa.*

Wide angle tomography, i.e. more than 10° allows visualization of the structures. Using this technique layers as thin as 1 mm can be imaged. Disadvantage of this technique is obtaining images of decreased contrast. Wide angle tomography is most useful when tissues of greater physical density such as bone are studied.

Narrow angle tomography uses an angle of less than 10° called *Zonography.*

STEREOSCOPY

It was introduced in 1898 by J Davidson. Stereoscopic imaging requires the exposure of two films one for each eye, and thus delivers twice the amount of radiation to the patient. Between exposures the patient is maintained in position, the film is changed and the tube is shifted from the right eye to the lift eye position. After processing the films commonly are viewed with a stereoscope that convergence of the viewer's eyes so that the brain can fuse the two images.

Indications

- To evaluate bony pockets in patient with periodontal disease
- Determination of root configuration of teeth that require endodontic therapy.
- Assessment of the relationship between mandibular canals to the roots of unerupted mandibular 3rd molars.
- Assessment of bone shape when placement of dental implants considered.
- To determine the location of small intracranial calcification and multiple foreign bodies in thick body sections.
- To evaluate the relationships of margins of bony fractures.

SCANOGRAPHY

It is a technique that used a narrow collimated, fan-shaped beam of radiation to scan an area of interest on to a moving film much same as in panoramic radiography. Scanograms demonstrate higher contrast because collimation of the X-ray beam reduces the amount of scattered radiation to the film during exposure.

Two types of scanography:

1. Rotational
2. Linear.

In *rotational scanography*, the beam of radiation rotates about a fixed axis that is predetermined based on the area to be imaged. X-ray tube is positioned differently to get a multiple images in which any two can be viewed as stereoscopic pairs. It is used in the assessment of periodontal disease and the detection of periapical lesions.

In *linear scanography*, X-ray beam and film move in a linear fashion, scanning the area of interest.

DIGITAL IMAGING

The application of computer technology to radiography has allowed image acquisition, manipulation, storage, retrieval and transmission to remote sites in a digital format.

- The use of digital technology results in 50–95% reduction in patient radiation exposure because of the greater sensitivity of the digital receptor.
- Elimination of film processing and no need of darkroom.
- Considerable reduction in the time lapse between image acquisition and display.

Digital imaging contains charge-coupled device (CCD) in the patient's mouth. After radiation exposure the signal from the CCD is sent to the computer where it is digitized into 256 gray levels. The image can then be displayed on a monitor, where it can be enhanced by varying the density and contrast. The image may also be stored for future use.

Digital radiography has two types:

1. Direct digital radiography
2. Indirect digital radiography.

Direct Digital Radiography

In direct digital radiography the image is acquired by some detector that is sensitive to electromagnetic energy either in the range of visible light or X-ray, then this data converted in to digitized form.

The following detectors are used to acquire an image:

- Photostimulable phosphor or storage phosphor plate (PSP)
- Charge-coupled device sensor (CCD)
- Complementary metal oxide semiconductor (CMOS)
- Flat panel detector

The PSP have X-ray absorption mechanisms similar to those of phosphors used in intensifying screens. The interaction between X-ray photons and crystals of PSP excites the electrons in the phosphor. Some of these electrons produce visible light in the usual manner but significant proportions are trapped within the phosphor.

When the phosphor subsequently is stimulated by irradiation with ruby laser, the trapped electrons are released, causing emission of shorter wavelength light in the blue region of the spectrum. The intensity of the emitted blue light is proportional to the amount of X-rays absorbed by the phosphor is detected by photomultiplier tube. The output of the tube is digitized to form the image.

Another type of detector is CCD. CCD consists of chip of pure silicon. When X-rays interact with the CCD an electric charge is created. The total electric charge developed and stored by a CCD is proportional to the X-ray energy absorbed. After the exposure of the CCD to radiation, electric charges are sequentially removed electronically creating an analog output signal by connecting to the computer where the acquired image can be manipulated.

Indirect Digital Radiography

In indirect digital radiography, radiographic film used as image receptor, the image is digitized from either video camera or CCD scanner or a laser scanner to view the radiographic image.

Indirect digital radiography results in less of information because the data acquired indirectly by the film results in reducing contrast and resolution of the image.

Advantages of Digital Radiography

- Eliminates the X-ray film so that reduces the cost of the film.
- It serves as recording, display and storage for diagnostic images.
- It requires less exposure time because of the greater sensitivity of the digital receptor thereby preventing patient from being exposed to radiation.
- Eliminates the chemical processing and dark room so that prevent the cause of allergy and pollution and also considerable reduction in time lapse between image acquisition and display.
- Film contrast, density, brightness and color may be manipulated so that increases the image information.
- Reduce the number of images that need to be remade because of over exposure or underexposure.
- Transmission (Teleradiography) of image to remote sites in a digital format.
- Image can be viewed on computer monitor and get a printout on paper.

Disadvantages

- Equipment is expensive
- Trained persons required to image acquisition and manipulation on computer.
- Patients have discomfort to keep bulky sensor inside the mouth.

Uses of Digital Radiography

- It can be used to view the image where multiple images required for analyzing.
- In endodontic practice to measure the root canal length, working length and distance between obturating material and the root apex.
- In periodontics, to assess and measure the height of the alveolar bone.
- Patient is uncooperative for regular radiographic techniques.
- To evaluate the bony changes in pathology of Jaws.
- To detection of initials dental caries.

COMPUTED TOMOGRAPHY

In 1972, *Godfrey Hounsfield* invented this technique and he referred as "Computerized axial transverse scanning (CAT scanning)" currently the preferred name is computed tomography or CT scan.

CT scan consists of a radiographic tube that emits a finely collimated fan shaped X-ray beam is directed to a series of scintillation detectors or ionization chambers. Both the radiographic tube and detectors may rotate synchronously about the patient; signal from the X-ray beam can be recorded by the scintillation detectors. These data can be fed into the computer where reconstruction of image can be made by data obtained from multiple projections.

The CT image is recorded and displayed as a matrix of individual blocks called *voxels*. Each square of the image matrix is a *pixel*.

Advantages

- This eliminates the superimposition of images of structures superficial or deep to the area of interest.
- Provides high contrast and resolution of images.
- CT distinguishes the tissues that differ in physical density by less than 1%. Where as conventional radiography requires 10% difference in physical density to distinguish between tissues.
- CT image provides multiple views as axial, coronal and sagittal sections depending on the diagnostic task.

Disadvantages

- Cost of the machine is high.
- Trained persons required.
- Large doses of irradiation cause biological effects in the body.

Uses of CT

- CT has a excellent diagnostic tool.
- Useful in the diagnosis of disease in the maxillofacial complex including salivary glands and TMJ.
- To evaluate the patient before placement of endosseous oral implant
- To view the cross-sectional images of entire maxilla and mandible.

MAGNETIC RESONANCE IMAGING

Magnetic resonance imaging (MRI) uses nonionizing radiation from the radiofrequency band of the electromagnetic spectrum.

The patient is placed inside a large magnet, which induces a strong external magnetic field causes the nuclei of many atoms in the body including hydrogen, to align themselves with the magnetic field. After application of radiofrequency signal, energy is released from the atoms that can be detected and used to construct the image by computer.

Advantages

- High sensitivity to detect tissue differences.
- No radiation exposure hence no radiation effects to the body.
- Excellent imaging techniques especially for soft tissue.
- It gives the best resolution of tissues of low inherent contrast.

Disadvantages

- Long imaging times
- It gives the potential hazard in a patient with implanted metallic foreign objects like, cardiac pacemakers, cerebral aneurysm clips.
- Some patients suffer from claustrophobia when positioned in a MRI machine.

Indications

- Diagnosing a suspected internal derangement of the TMJ
- Postsurgical evaluation of TMJ.
- Identifying and localizing orofacial soft tissue lesions.
- Provides the image of salivary gland parenchyma.

NUCLEAR MEDICINE OR RADIONUCLIDE IMAGING OR SCINTIGRAPHY

Nuclear medicine is based on the radiotracer method. Radioactive atoms or molecules in organs behave in a manner identical to that of other molecules in the body and they are chemically indistinguishable. This radiotracers allow measurement of tissue function and provide early marker of disease through measurement of biochemical change in tissues before any physical signs and symptoms occurs.

Radioactive substances should be injected intravenously into the patient and rectilinear scanner or gamma scintillation camera records the gamma emission from the patient. The camera uses a scintillation crystal that has the ability to fluoresce on interaction with gamma rays emitting from the radioactive substance. This emitting light (fluorescence) is detected by a photomultiplier tube that magnifies and amplifies the signals many times to produce an image.

Many gamma emitting isotopes have been used in radionuclide imaging including iodine, gallium, selenium and most commonly used technetium known as *technetium pertechnetate (99mTc)*.

Recent developments in nuclear medicines are:

- SPECT scan (single photon emission computed tomography
- PET scan (positron emission tomography)

In this technique either multiple detectors or a single moving detector which records the data in a different section obtained from the radioactive substance which emits the gamma rays injected into the patient's body.

Advantages

- Radionuclide imaging is much more sensitive to early or small changes in bone or salivary gland metabolism.
- It has been used to detect the presence and size of tumors, metastasis, osteo-arthrosis, trauma and metabolic disorders.

Disadvantages

- Poor, grainy image.
- Confusion of normal inflammatory process with tumor and metastasis.
- Patient also exposed to small quantity of radioactive materiel, which causes biological changes in the tissues.

ULTRASONOGRAPHY OR SONOGRAPHY

The sound can be audible if it lies between 1500 and 20,000 cycles/sec (Hertz-Hz). In ultrasound frequency vibration is greater than 20 K Hz which is more than the audible range. In diagnostic sonography, ultrasound used in the frequency of 1–20 MHz. Scanners used for sonography generate electrical impulses that are connected into ultra-high frequency sound waves by a transducer, which is a device that can convert electrical energy into sound energy.

The most important component of the transducer is a thin *piezo*-electric crystals or material made up of a great number of dipoles arranged in a geometric pattern. A dipole may have a positive charge on one end and a negative charge on the other. The electrical impulse generated by the scanner causes the dipoles in the crystal to realign themselves with the electrical field and thus suddenly change the crystal's thickness. These abrupt changes being a series of vibrations that produce the sound waves that are transmitted into the tissues being examined.

When ultrasonic beam passes through or interacts with tissues of different sound energy obstruction, reflection, refraction and diffusion. Sonic waves that reflected back (Echoed) toward the transducer cause a change in the thickness of the piezoelectric crystal, which produces an electrical signal that is amplified, processed and displayed on a monitor. In this system the transducer serves as both a transmitter and a receiver.

Ultrasonography useful in detecting the soft tissue pathology especially in the TMJ and abdomen.

ELECTRONIC THERMOGRAPHY

The uses of thermography in diagnosis are based on the fact that diseases and abnormal conditions may result in different temperature patterns because of alterations in blood supply or the presence of inflammation. Sensors used to record temperature differences are displayed as a color image on a video monitor. Color differences may represent temperature changes as little as 0.1°C. It is useful in diagnosing diseases of the maxillofacial complex, determining tooth's vitality; evaluate a case of atypical odontalgia and internal derangement of the TMJ.

ARTHROGRAPHY

It is technique in which image of the TMJ disc is obtained by injecting a radiopaque contrast agent into one or both joint spaces and sequential radiographs are taken.

Arthrography is indicated when information about disc position, function, morphology and treatment planning.

This procedure is contraindicated when the patient is allergic to iodine contrast agent and risk of infection.

XERORADIOGRAPHY

Xeroradiography is an imaging technique that has been proposed as an alternative to conventional X-ray film radiography.

In xeroradiography, the X-ray image is recorded on a photoconductive selenium coated plate rather than X-ray film, selenium coated plate is charged and placed into a light tight cassette. This photoreceptor is placed intraorally and exposed to X-ray beam causing selective discharge. The amount of discharge related to amount of radiation striking the photoreceptor.

During developing, the selenium plate is exposed to a cloud of charged powder particles called toner. Individual toner particles are attracted to the charged plate and deposited on the plate to develop the image.

Next the plate is dried to remove the liquid vehicle of toner particles. The processed image is transferred on to clear adhesive tape and fixed to an opaque plastic base. The resulting image may be viewed either as a photograph with reflected light or as a radiograph with transmitted light from a view box.

Advantages

- Reduction in exposure time
- Wide latitude of exposure
- Ease in manipulation
- Ease of viewing
- Elimination of accidental film exposure.
- Superior edge contrast.

Disadvantages

- Patient discomfort
- Cost of the machine is high
- Slower speed.

SIALOGRAPHY

It is a specialized radiographic technique in which radiopaque contrast media is injected into the ducts of the salivary grand and visualized through radiographs taken sequentially.

Indications

- Detection of calculus (Sialolith) or foreign bodies in the duct or in the parenchymal tissue of salivary glands.
- Detection of fistula, diverticulum in the salivary glands.
- Detection and diagnosis of recurrent swelling in inflammatory process.
- Demonstration of tumor and its location, size and origin.

Contraindications

- It cannot be used in patient with sensitivity to iodine compounds.
- In acute inflammation of salivary glands.
- Residual iodine contrast media might interfere with subsequent thyroid test.

Contrast Media

Contrast media are radiopaque substances that are introduced in to different parts of the body to alter subject contrast artificially **(Table 10.1)**. Contrast media used for sialography are divided into:

- Water-soluble, for example
  - Conray 480
  - Hypaque
  - Renografin
  - Sinografin
  - Isopaque
  - Triosil
- Fat-soluble, for example
  - Ethiodol
  - Lipiodol

Advantages and disadvantages of water and fat-soluble contrast agents are tabulated in **Table 10.2**.

Table 10.1: Different radiographic techniques are performed by using contrast media

Radiographic technique	*Tissue or organs*
Sialography	Salivary glands
Arthrography	Joints
Angiography	Blood vessels
Lymphography	Lymph nodes and vessels
Urography	Kidneys
Barium meal	Stomach and duodenum
Contrast computed tomography	General enhancement
Contrast MRI	Tissue enhancement

Table 10.2: Advantages and disadvantages of contrast agents

Contrast agents	*Advantages*	*Disadvantages*
Water soluble	• Low viscosity, thus easily introduced • Easily and rapidly removed from the gland	• Less radiopaque thus show reduced contrast • Short time retain in the gland
Fat soluble	• Dense radiopaque, thus show good contrast • High viscosity, thus slow excretion from the gland	• Long time retain in the gland produce foreign body reaction • It does not flow easily into the gland

Properties of Contrast Media

- It should have physiological properties similar to saliva.
- Absence of local or systemic toxicity.
- Satisfactory radiopaque.
- Low surface tension and viscosity allow filling of the fine components of ductal system.

Sialographic Technique

The technique is divided into three phases:

1. Preoperative phase
2. The filling phase
3. The emptying phase.

Preoperative phase: This involves taking preoperative (scout) radiographs before the introduction of the contrast media to know the position and presence of any obstruction and also to assess the position of shadow cast that may overlie the gland.

Filling phase: After obtaining the scout films, and insert the cannula slowly into the dilated duct orifice and introduce the contrast media into the ductal system until the patient experiences tightness or discomfort in the gland (about 0.7 mL for parotid gland, 0.5 mL for submandibular gland).

Emptying phase: The cannula is removed and the patient allowed rinsing with lemon juice aid to excretion of the contrast media. After the emptying phase lateral oblique view of mandible radiographs are taken. Sialographic appearances of normal parotid gland:

Branching duct structure regularly and tapers gradually towards periphery of the gland appeared as a *"tree-in-winter"* **(Figs 10.2A and B)**

Sialographic Appearances of Normal Submandibular Gland

This gland is smaller than parotid but overall picture shows similar findings as in parotid, so called *"bush-in-winter"* **(Figs 10.3A and B)**.

Sialographic Appearances of Salivary Calculi

- Filling defect in the main duct.
- Ductal dilatation caused by infection.
- Contrast media retain behind the stone.

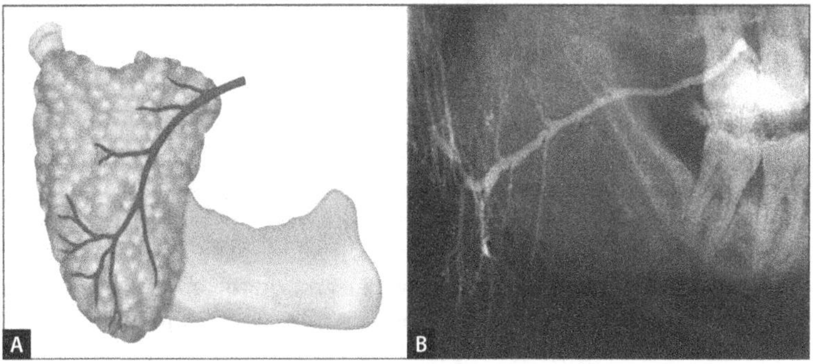

Figs 10.2A and B: Normal appearance of parotid gland and duct on sialography as a tree-in-winter or leafless tree. (A) Schematic diagram of parotid gland appearance on sialography; (B) Lateral view of parotid gland appearance on sialography

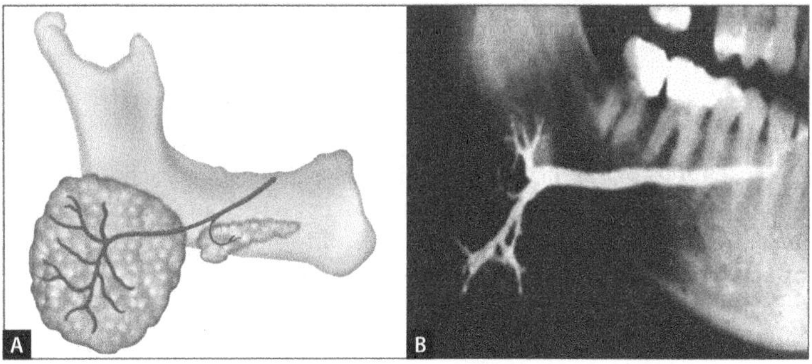

Figs 10.3A and B: Normal appearance of submandibular gland on sialography as a bush-in-winter appearance; (A) Schematic diagram of submandibular gland appearance on sialography; (B) Lateral view of submandibular gland appearance on sialography

Sialographic Appearances of Sialadenitis

- Dots or blobs of contrast media within the gland producing dilatation of the acini.
- The main duct is normal.

Sialographic Appearances of Sjögren's Syndrome

Widespread dots or blobs of contrast media within the gland appeared as a snow storm.

CONE BEAM COMPUTED TOMOGRAPHY

Cone beam computed tomography [(CBCT), also referred to as C-arm CT, cone beam volume CT, or flat panel CT] is a medical imaging technique consisting of X-ray computed tomography where the X-rays are divergent, forming a cone.

Imaging is accomplished by using a rotating gantry to which an X-ray source and detector are fixed. A divergent pyramidal- or cone-shaped source of ionizing radiation is directed through the middle of the area of interest onto an area X-ray detector on the opposite side. The X-ray source and detector rotate around a rotation fulcrum fixed within the center of the region of interest. During the rotation, multiple (from 150 to more than 600) sequential planar projection images of the field of view (FOV) are acquired in a complete, or sometimes partial, arc.

CBCT image production can be explained under three steps:
1. Acquisition configuration.
2. Image reconstruction.
3. Image display.

Image Acquisition

X-rays penetrate the patient from different angles and reach the image receptor (usually flat panel detector). These receptors measure the amount of X-rays penetrating the patient from various angles and this process is known as image acquisition.

Image Reconstruction

Once these attenuated X-rays reach the image receptor, they are transferred to the computer. Here the software, mathematically calculates the attenuated X-ray information and produces a CT image volume. This process is known as image reconstruction.

Image Display

After the image reconstruction, the computer will enable the display of the image in axial, sagittal, coronal sections and 3D format using any image viewing software. These images are displayed in DICOM format (Digital Imaging and Communications in Medicine).

Field of View

The dimensions of the FOV or scan volume able to be covered depend primarily on the detector size and shape, the beam projection geometry,

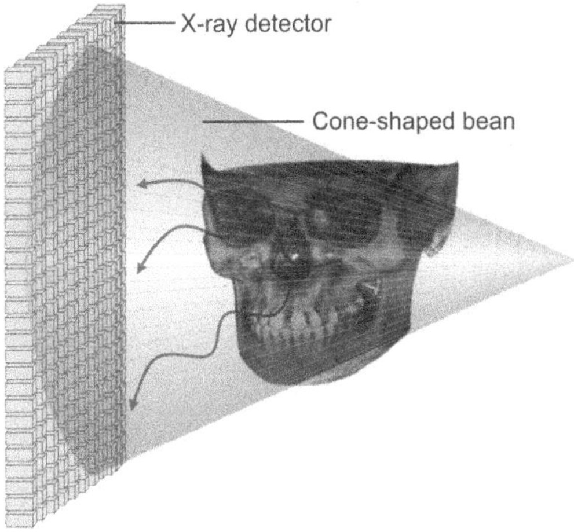

Fig. 10.4: Cone-shaped X-ray beam in CBCT imaqe production

and the ability to collimate the beam. The shape of the scan volume can be either cylindrical or spherical **(Fig. 10.4)**. Collimation of the primary X-ray beam limits X-radiation exposure to the region of interest. Field size limitation therefore ensures that an optimal FOV can be selected for each patient, based on disease presentation and the region designated to be imaged. CBCT systems can be categorized according to the available FOV or selected scan volume height as follows:

- *Localized region:* Approximately 5 cm or less (e.g. dentoalveolar, temporomandibular joint)
- *Single arch:* 5–7 cm (e.g. maxilla or mandible)
- *Interarch:* 7–10 cm (e.g. mandible and superiorly to include the inferior concha)
- *Maxillofacial:* 10–15 cm (e.g. mandible and extending to Nasion)
- *Craniofacial:* Greater than 15 cm (e.g. from the lower border of the mandible to the vertex of the head)
- Extended FOV scanning incorporating the craniofacial region is difficult to incorporate into cone-beam design because of the high cost of large-area.

Image Receptors in CBCT

Image receptors in CBCT are of four types:

1. Image intensifier coupled to charge-coupled device (IIT/CCD)
2. Complementary metal oxide semiconductor (CMOS)

3. Thin film transistor (TFT)
4. Flat-panel detectors (FPD)

Most of the presently marketed CBCT machines either use TFT or FPD type of image receptors.

Artifacts

The common artifacts seen in CBCT images are:

- Beam hardening
- Metal artefacts
- Radiographic noise
- Motion artifact
- Exomass.

Uses of CBCT

The current applications of CBCT appear to have impacted all the specialties of dentistry:

- Evaluation of implant placement, position and postimplant status
- Inferior alveolar nerve and sinus floor location
- Assessment of impacted teeth position
- Paranasal sinus evaluation
- Presurgical implant site assessment
- Odontogenic lesion visualization
- Endodontic diagnoses
- Diagnosis of temporomandibular joint disorders
- Other CAD/CAM devices (3D models)
- Trauma evaluation.

Advantages

- Rapid scan time
- Beam limitation
- *Image accuracy:* Capable of providing accurate, submillimeter-resolution images in formats allowing 3D visualization of the complexity of the maxillofacial region.
- Reduced patient radiation dose
- Interactive display modes applicable to maxillofacial imaging
- Multiplanar reformation
- Ray sum or ray casting
- Three-dimensional volume rendering
- Indirect volume rendering.
- Direct volume rendering

Limitations of CBCT

There are some important limitations of CBCT are:

- Inability to give details of soft tissues.
- CBCT machine produces more scatter radiation than the medical CT machines. Majority of the machines provide antiscatter software algorithms.
- Some of the CBCT machines need to be calibrated more often and this can reduce the productivity of the busy radiology department.
- Hounsfield units measured in a CBCT unit are yet to be proven as reliable data for the determination of the bone quality.

CHAPTER 11

Infection Control in Radiography

Dental personnel and patients are at increased risk of acquiring tuberculosis, herpes infection, upper respiratory infections hepatitis, and acquired immune deficiency syndrome (AIDS).

Human blood and saliva are known to be infectious for hepatitis and human immunodeficiency virus (HIV). The main rationale in infection control is to block the transmission of infectious agents between patients and dental personnel or other patients.

Dental radiography is normally a noninvasive investigation. Therefore, the risk of cross infection from one patient to another or to dental personnel is usually only from salivary contamination. However, appropriate precautions against cross infection should be taken for all patients.

Latex rubber gloves should be worn. Gloved hands should be washed before and after X-raying every patient, with soap and water, then rinse and dry them and apply a disinfectant.

All film holders; bite blocks should be rinsed before and after use, then sterilized by autoclaving.

Saliva should be wiped from exposed film before processing.

X-ray equipment, including tube head, control panel timer and cassettes should be wiped with a suitable disinfectant (Sodium hypochlorite).

SOURCES OF INFECTION

Everything that we touch during radiographic procedures is a possible transmitter of pathogens. A pathogen is a microorganism that can cause disease. The most common pathogens that can be transmitted in the dental office include:

- Infective hepatitis caused by hepatitis B (HBV) or hepatitis C (HCV) viruses.
- Human immunodeficiency virus (HIV disease and AIDS caused by HIV)
- Tuberculosis (TB)
- Cold sores caused by herpes simplex virus (HSV). Healthcare workers are at risk of getting herpetic whitlow, a painful finger infection.

- Rubella (German measles)
- Syphilis
- Diphtheria
- Mumps
- Influenza
- Transmissible spongiform encephalopathies (TSEs).

The X-ray machine, the control panel and exposure switch, clothing, counter tops, the dental chair, the light handle, walls, door knobs, processors, and patient records. In short, any object that the operator touches after placing the packet in the patient's mouth can be considered contaminated and a source of transmission to the operator or other patients. Any object that is touched before working in the mouth can be considered a source of transmission to the patient. Thus barriers (*universal barriers*) to the transmission of infective microorganisms must be used. Barriers include gloves, masks, protective eyewear, gowns and surface coverings.

Infection control in dental radiography can be broadly classified under four headings:

1. Infection control procedures used before exposure
2. Infection control procedures used during exposure
3. Infection control procedures used after exposure
4. Infection control procedures used for processing.

INFECTION CONTROL PROCEDURES EMPLOYED BEFORE EXPOSURE

Before dental X-ray films are exposed, the treatment area must be prepared using aseptic technique. Necessary supplies and equipment must also be prepared.

Preparation of the Treatment Area

The dental professional must prepare the surfaces that are likely to be touched during the X-ray exposure should be covered with impervious, disposable materials such as plastic-wrap, plastic-backed paper, or aluminum foil. Covering the exposed surfaces with such disposable materials provides adequate protection while eliminating the need for surface cleaning and disinfection between patients.

Examples of surfaces that must be covered or disinfected include:
X-ray machine: The tube-head, PID, control panel and exposure button must be covered or disinfected using suitable surface disinfectant, e.g. Mikrozid **(Figs 11.1A and B)**.

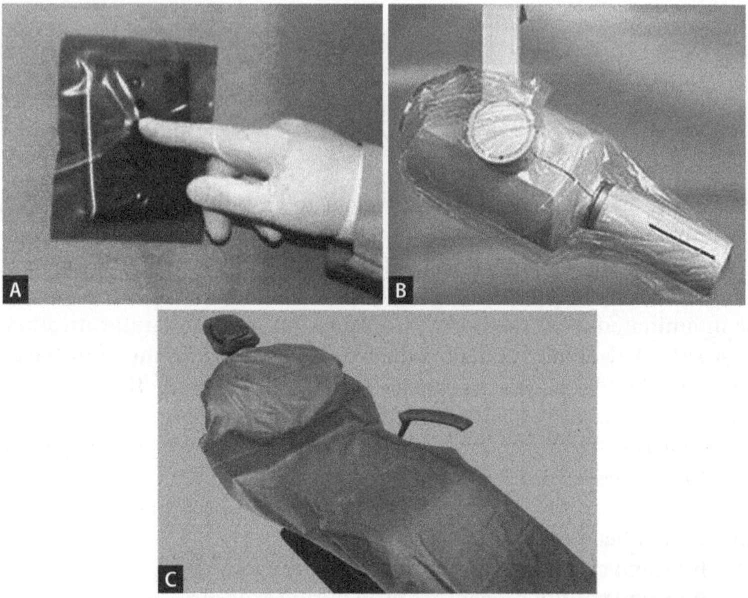

Figs 11.1A to C: (A) X-ray control panel covered with barrier; (B) Plastic wrapped around X-ray tube; (C) Plastic barrier to X-ray chair

Dental chair: The headrest, headrest adjustment, and chair adjustment controls must all be covered or disinfected using suitable surface disinfectant, e.g. Mikrozid **(Fig. 11.1C)**.

Work area: The area where X-ray supplies (e.g. film) are placed during exposure must be covered or disinfected using suitable surface disinfectant, e.g. Mikrozid.

Lead apron: If contaminated, the lead apron must be wiped with a disinfectant between patients.

Preparation of Supplies and Equipment

The dental professional must also prepare all anticipated supplies and equipment, such as film, sterilized film-holding devices, and other miscellaneous items, and must make these available in the work area.

Film: Dental X-ray films should be dispensed from a central supply area in a disposable container (e.g. coin envelope, paper cup). Commercially available *plastic barrier envelopes* that fit over intraoral films can be used

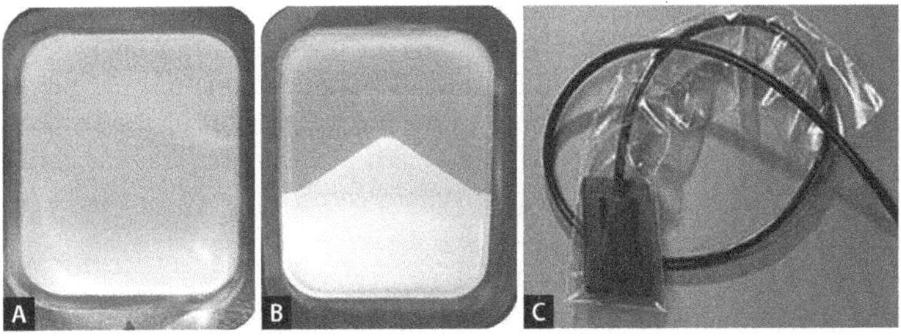

Figs 11.2A to C: (A) Commercially available intraoral periapical film sealed in plastic barrier (front or tube side); (B) Backside of film in plastic barrier; (C) Digital sensor with barrier envelopes

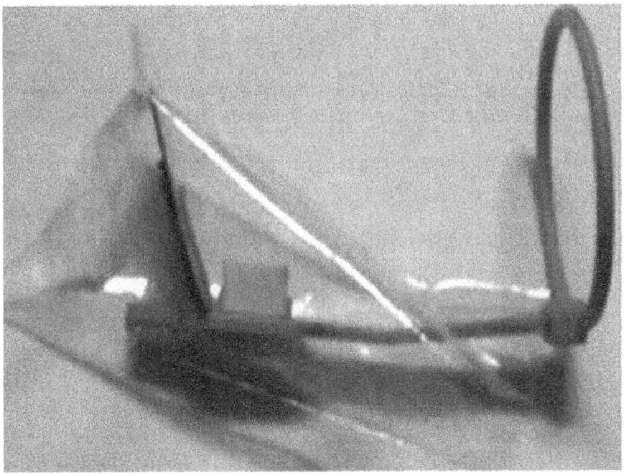

Fig. 11.3: X-ray film (XCP) holder with film wrapped with plastic barrier

to protect the film packets from saliva and minimize contamination after exposure of the film. Intraoral films may be inserted and sealed in plastic barrier envelopes **(Figs 11.2A and B)** (e.g. Clin-Asept Barrier Envelopes manufactured by Kodak) before dispensing films from a central supply area. Digital radiography sensors must also be placed inside appropriate barrier envelopes **(Fig. 11.2C)**.

Film-holding devices: They should be packaged in sterilized bags and dispensed from a central supply area. Disposable film-holding devices can also be used **(Fig. 11.3)**.

Miscellaneous items: Other items include cotton rolls that can be used to stabilize the film placement and paper towels that can be used to remove saliva from exposed films. A disposable container (e.g. paper cup) labeled with patient's name is also necessary to collect the exposed films. All miscellaneous items should also be dispensed from a central supply area.

Preparation of the Patient

The dental professional can seat the patient following preparation of the treatment area, supplies and equipment. After seating the patient, the dental radiographer must complete the following procedures.

Chair adjustment: The chair must be positioned so that the patient is seated upright. The height of the chair should be adjusted to a comfortable working height for the dental radiographer.

Headrest adjustment: The headrest must be adjusted to support the patient's head. The patient's head should be positioned with the upper arch parallel to the floor.

Lead apron: The lead apron with the thyroid collar must be placed on the patient and secured before any X-ray exposure.

Miscellaneous objects: Miscellaneous objects belonging to the patient that may interfere with film exposure (e.g. eyeglasses, chewing gum, dentures) must be removed by the patient at this time.

Preparation of the Dental Radiographer

After patient preparation and before X-ray exposure of the patient, the dental radiographer must complete some final infection control procedures.

Handwashing: Hands must be washed with some soap or an antimicrobial solution in the presence of the patient.

Gloves: Immediately after handwashing, gloves must be placed **(Fig. 11.4)**.

Mask and eyewear: Because no aerosolized contamination is created during radiographic exposures, the use of a surgical mask and protective eyewear is optional.

Film-holding devices: If film-holding devices are to be used during exposure, then they must be removed from sterilized packages with gloved hands in the presence of the patient and then assembled.

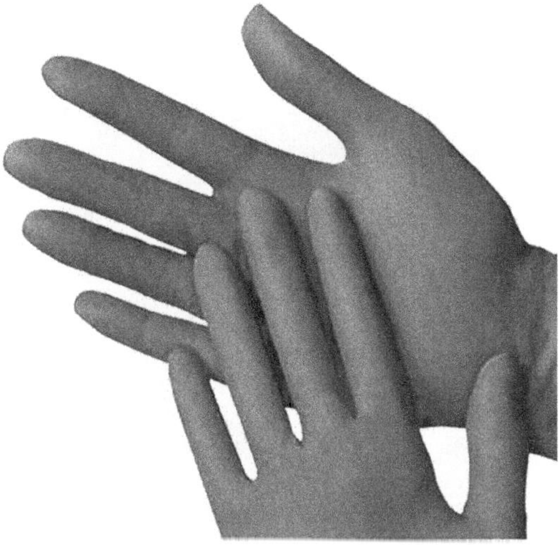

Fig. 11.4: Hand gloves must wear before any radiological procedures

INFECTION CONTROL PROCEDURES USED DURING EXPOSURE

Once gloves have been put on and exposure of X-ray films begins, the dental radiographer should take special care to touch only covered surfaces. The best way the dental radiographer can minimize contamination is to touch as few surfaces as possible. During and immediately after film exposure, the dental radiographer must handle each film in a manner consistent with comprehensive infection control guidelines.

Drying of exposed films: After each film has been placed in the patient's mouth, exposed, and removed, it must be dried with a paper towel to remove excess saliva. Saliva can also be wiped off from exposed film packets with 1% hypochlorite disinfectant.

Collection of exposed films: Once dried, each film must be placed in a disposable container (paper bag or paper cup) labeled with the patient's name. This container is used to collect and transport the exposed films to the darkroom and must not be touched by gloved hands **(Fig. 11.5)**. To prevent film fog caused by scattered radiation, the container should not be placed in a room where additional films are being exposed. In addition, exposed films should never be placed in the dental radiographer's laboratory coat or uniform pocket.

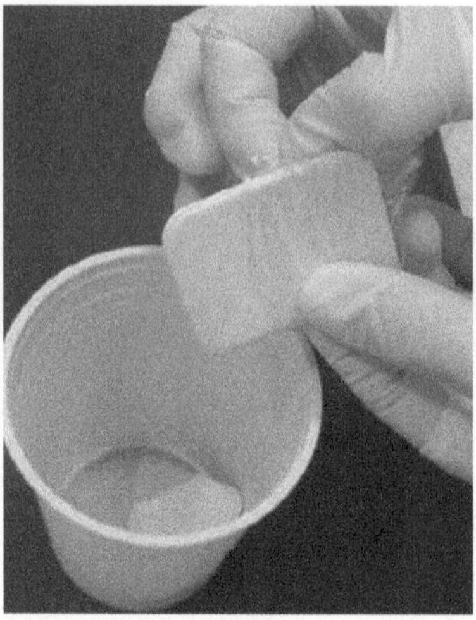

Fig. 11.5: Plastic barrier removed over the film carefully without touching the film with contaminated gloves

Film-holding devices: During exposures, film-holding devices should be transferred from the covered work area to the patient's mouth and then back to the same area. Contaminated instruments should never be placed on an uncovered countertop.

Interruptions during exposure: If the dental radiographer is interrupted and must leave the room during exposure of films (e.g. in response to a telephone call), gloves must be removed and hands must be washed before leaving the area. The hands must then be rewashed and new gloves put on before resuming with exposures.

INFECTION CONTROL PROCEDURES USED AFTER EXPOSURE

Immediately after the completion of film exposures, all contaminated items must be discarded, and any uncovered areas must be disinfected.

Disposal of contaminated items: All contaminated material (cotton rolls, bitewing tabs, cups, bags, and protective coverings) must be properly disposed. The dental radiographer must carefully un-wrap all covered surfaces. Ideally, the disposal of all contaminated items should take place in the presence of the patient.

Film-holding devices: While the dental radiographer is wearing gloves, the contaminated film-holding devices must be removed from the treatment area and placed in an area designated for contaminated instruments.

Handwash: After removal and disposal of all contaminated items, the gloves must be removed and discarded and hands must be washed.

Lead apron removal: After the hands have been washed, the lead apron can be removed from the patient. At this time, the patient can be dismissed from the X-ray area.

Surface disinfection: Any uncovered areas that were contaminated during treatment must be cleaned and disinfected using suitable surface disinfectant, e.g. Mikrozid.

INFECTION CONTROL PROCEDURES USED FOR PROCESSING

After exposure of X-ray films, specific infection control guidelines must be followed during transport of the films to the darkroom, during film handling, and during film processing.

Film transport: As previously described, films contaminated with saliva must be placed in a labeled disposable container after exposure. The disposable container should never be touched by a gloved hand. Only after the gloves have been removed, the hands have been washed, the patient has been dismissed, and the area has been cleaned, should the dental radiographer carry the disposable container holding the contaminated films to the darkroom.

Darkroom supplies: Paper towels and gloves are necessary for film handling before processing and must be available in the darkroom. Paper envelopes, paper cups, or film mounts, labeled with patient's name, and used to hold the films after processing **(Fig. 11.6)** should be available in the darkroom.

Disinfection of the darkroom: Darkroom countertops should be disinfected properly.

Film-handling with or without barrier envelopes: Commercially available barrier envelopes help to minimize contamination in the darkroom. **Table 11.1** lists the recommended film-handling steps when exposed films are protected by barrier envelopes and when films are not protected by barrier envelopes.

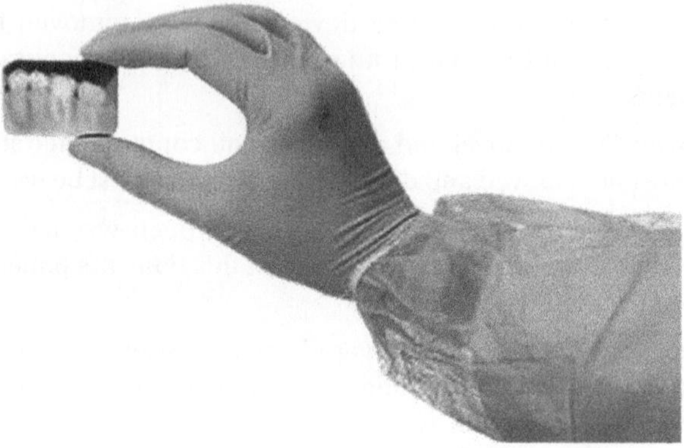

Fig. 11.6: Film should be held with gloves after processing

Daylight Loader Procedures

Infection control procedures for processing films without barrier envelopes in automatic film processors equipped with daylight loaders include the following:

- Place paper cup and vinyl or non-powdered gloves in daylight loader compartment (Powdered gloves may cause artifacts on the films).
- Place container with contaminated films next to cup.
- Close daylight loader lid and push hands through openings.
- Put on gloves.
- Take one contaminated film out of container.
- Open film packets as described in film handling without barrier envelopes **(Table 11.1)**.
- Allow film to drop onto processor film feed slot area (Do not touch film with gloved hands).
- Dispose the film packet wrappings in the paper cup.
- After all film packets have been opened, remove gloves and place in cup.
- Feed all unwrapped films into processor.
- Remove hands from daylight loader.
- Wash hands.
- Lift daylight loader lid to remove and discard cup with contaminated wrappings and container that held contaminated films.
- Label a film mount, paper cup, or envelope with the patient's name, and use to collect processed films.

Table 11.1: Steps for film handling during processing

I. With barrier envelopes
• Place disposable towel on work surface in darkroom • Place container with contaminated films next to towel • Put on gloves • Take one contaminated film out of container • Tear open barrier envelope • Allow film to drop on paper towel • Do not touch film with gloved hands • Dispose of barrier envelope • After all barrier envelopes have been opened, dispose of container • Remove gloves and wash hands • Turn out darkroom lights and secure door • Unwrap and process films • Label a film mount, paper cup, or envelope with the patient's name, and use to collect processed films
II. Without barrier envelopes (Fig. 11.7)
• Place disposable towel on work surface in darkroom • Place container with contaminated films next to towel • Put on gloves • Turn out darkroom lights and secure door • Take one contaminated film out of container • Open film packet tab and slide out lead foil backing and black paper. Discard film packet wrapping • Rotate foil away from black paper and discard • Without touching the film, open the black paper wrapping • Allow film to drop on paper towel • Do not touch film with gloved hands • Discard black paper wrapping • After all barrier envelopes have been opened, dispose of container • Remove gloves and wash hands. • Process films • Label a film mount, paper cup, or envelope with the patient's name, and use to collect processed films

Infection Control in Panoramic X-ray Units

Because panoramic radiography is an extra-oral procedure, fewer areas are contaminated by the patient's saliva. The patient bite block should be covered by a plastic barrier cover or autoclavable, if possible. Plastic barrier wrap should be used on the chin rest, ear rods, and patient handgrips. Processing presents no problems because the cassette does not contact the patient; thus the procedure for preventing film contamination is not necessary.

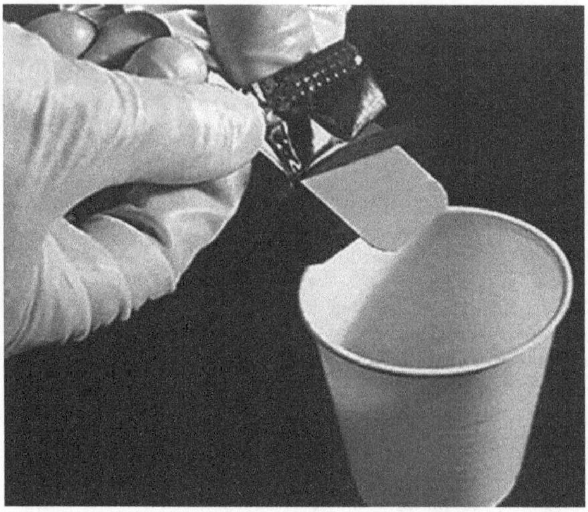

Fig. 11.7: Unwrapped film carefully without touching the film with gloves

Cephalostat ear rods, forehead supporter and nasion pointer can be disinfected by wiping with an iodine-detergent solutions. These may covered in plastic after cleaning.

CHAPTER 12

Radiographic Interpretation of Lesions

Interpretation of radiographs is to uncovering all the information contained within the black, white and gray radiographic images.

The main objectives are:

- To identify the presence or absence of disease.
- To provide information on the nature and extent of the disease.
- To enable the formation of a differential diagnosis.

To achieve these objectives and maximize the diagnostic yield, interpretation should be carried out under specified conditions and systematic guidelines.

ESSENTIAL REQUIREMENTS FOR INTERPRETATION

The essential requirements for interpreting dental radiographs can be summarized as follows:

- Optimum viewing conditions.
- Understanding of the nature of black, white and gray radiographic image.
- Detailed knowledge of the radiographical appearances of normal anatomical structures.
- Detailed knowledge of the radiographic appearances of the diseases.

The image is produced by X-rays passing through an object and interacting with the photographic emulsion on a film. This interaction results in blackening of the film. The extent to which the emulsion is blackened depends on the number of X-rays reaching the film which in turn depends on the density of the object.

The white or radiopaque shadows on the film represent the various dense structures within the object which have totally stopped the X-ray beam (e.g. enamel, dentine, cementum and alveolar bone).

The black or radiolucent shadows represent areas where the X-ray beam has passed through the object (e.g. pulp, periodontal space, marrow space and air space).

Aunt Minnie Approach

Aunt Minnie represents an abnormality which looks like one that the evaluator has seen before, or been told about. It would be difficult to recognize new findings using this approach.

Cousin Harry represents an abnormality which the evaluator has not seen for a long time, but would like to see.

Uncle Fred represents an abnormality which is often present.

A systematic radiological description of a lesion should include:
- Size
- Shape
- Location
- Borders or edge
- Relative radiodensity or internal structure
- Effects on adjacent structures.

Size

- Measure the lesion with a ruler and use surrounding structures as guide. Measure in two dimensions, width and height either in millimeter or centimeter.
- If impacted tooth having surrounding small radiolucent follicle is considered as normal, but larger follicle is likely to be considered as dentigerous cyst.
- Periapical cyst always have larger radiolucent lesion than periapical granuloma.

Shape

- Circular, fluid filled (hydraulic) are likely to be a cyst.
- Scalloped-multilocular lesion is referred to as odontogenic keratocyst.

Location

- *Soft tissue lesions:* If epicenter of the lesion coronal to tooth structure, commonly recognized as origin from odontogenic epithelium.
- *Bony lesions:*
  - Epicenter of the lesion is above the mandibular canal usually odontogenic in origin.
  - If epicenter below mandibular canal likely to be non-odontogenic.

- If epicenter from the canal itself likely to be neurovascular lesions.
- Cartilaginous lesions and osteochondroma are commonly located in the condyles.
- The central giant cell granuloma usually arises anterior to the first molar in mandible and canine in the maxilla.
- Osteomyelitis occurs in mandible region only.

Borders or Margins

- Any lesion either it could be well-defined or poorly or ill-defined border.
- Well-defined borders are one, a clear-cut demarcation between normal and abnormal bony structures.
- Well-defined borders are corticated or not corticated, sclerotic or not sclerotic and punched out borders.
- A corticated border is a thin, uniform radiopaque line of reactive bone at the edge of the lesion.
- Sclerotic border is a wide, radiopaque margin of reactive bone that usually not uniform in width. This may be seen in periapical cemental dysplasia and may indicate a very slow rate of growth.
- Radiopaque lesion may have soft tissue capsule surrounding the lesion, radiographically, it appears as radiolucent ring or halo. This is a characteristic sign found in odontoma and cementoblastoma.
- Punched out lesions is clear-cut delineation from the normal bone, usually found in multiple myeloma.
- Poorly defined lesions shows no delineation between normal and the abnormal bone, there is blending of margins. Sometime, it may invade into the normal bone as a finger-like projection. This type of border is usually seen in malignant lesions, where lesion is rapidly grows and spreads in to the surrounding healthy bone results in few trabeculae are lost and remaining trabeculae demonstrates poorly defined with finger-like projections.

Internal Structures

- Internal structure radiographically interpreted as either radiopaque or radiolucent and sometimes mixed lesion.
- Radiolucent structures are contains air, fat, gas, fluid, bone marrow and soft tissue.
- The appearance of radiopacity is due to their contents such as, trabecular bone, cortical bone, enamel, metal and calcified structures.

- Internal structures may have septae or loculations, these septae are residual bone with long strands/walls and loculations are individual compartments. If the lesion contains more than one compartment, usually known as "multilocular" and single compartment is "unilocular".
- If the compartments are uniform in width appears as "Honeycomb", and varying in size are known as "Soap bubble appearance". It may be seen in ameloblastoma, central hemangioma, central giant cell granuloma and odontogenic keratocyst.
- In odontogenic-myxoma and septa are appears as straight, thin as "Tennis racket" a unique characteristic features.

Effects on Adjacent Structure

- Widening of periodontal ligament is uniform or irregular, if widening occurs at periapical area associated with dental caries indicating periapical periodontitis or periapical abscess. If it is seen at the lateral part of the root region commonly identified as periodontal infection along with discontinuity of lamina dura.
- Widening of periodontal ligament space with absence of periapical or periodontal infection, suspected an early osteosarcomatous lesion.
- Displacement of teeth, mandibular canal, maxillary sinus and other anatomical structures commonly seen with slow growing tumor (benign tumor).
- In malignant lesions, due to rapid spreading of the lesion, it encroaches or invading into the surrounding structures such as tooth, mandibular canal, and maxillary sinus.
- Benign neurovascular lesions may widen the mandibular canal without destruction of cortical boundary, but destruction of cortical boundary of canal seen in the malignant neurovascular.
- Benign lesion may allow sufficient time for the outer periosteum to produce new bone so that bony expansion takes place without destruction of cortical plate.
- Due to rapid growth of malignant lesions produce destruction of cortical plate known as pathological fracture of bone.
- Different periosteal reactions occurs depending upon the severity of the lesion, produce different appearances such as onion-peel appearance, sunburst and Codman's triangle.

SYSTEMATIC ANALYSIS OF INTRAOSSEOUS LESION

Site or Location

Depending upon the site, assess the lesion originate from the odontogenic or nonodontogenic tissues.

Size

Slow-growing (benign) lesions have smaller in size unless any secondary changes such as inflammation. In contrast rapidly growing (malignant) lesions may have larger in size.

Shape

Slow-growing lesions always round or oval in shape, but irregular in shape occurs in rapidly growing lesions.

Borders or Periphery

Slow-growing or chronic lesions have well-defined borders, and cyst may have corticated borders. Poorly or ill-defined margin is seen in rapidly growing and acute lesions.

Internal Structures

Kind of lesions can be determined by its content that radiographically appears as:

- *Radiopaque:* Osteoblastic in nature (malignant lesions, secondary changes such as calcification and chronic cases of slow inflammatory [condensing osteitis] lesions).
- *Radiolucent:* Osteolytic in nature (benign lesions, cystic lesions, early stages of inflammatory lesions)
- *Mixed lesions:* Both osteoblastic and osteolytic in nature (intermediate stage of some benign [cementoma] lesions).

Effects on Surrounding Structures

- Displacement of tooth, mandibular canal, maxillary sinus.
- Periodontal ligament space widening and discontinuity of lamina dura.
- Outer cortical bone and periosteal reaction.

CHAPTER 13

Radiographic Interpretation of Dental Caries

The diagnosis of caries is made through a combination of the clinical examination and radiographs. Unless fairly large, interproximal caries in the posterior region usually requires radiographs to make a diagnosis.

The bitewing film is primarily used for caries identification, but the periapical film is also helpful. The difference in angulation between the two films gives two different perspectives, and can be especially helpful in diagnosing recurrent caries around existing restorations.

There is a lot of discussion on which film speed (D or F) should be used. Many dentists use D-speed film because they feel it provides sharper images as a result of the smaller grain size. Most educators, on the other hand, recommend the F-speed film (insight) because of the significant reduction in X-ray exposure to the patient (approximately 60% less than when using D-speed film).

Approximately, 40–50% demineralization is required for radiographic detection of a lesion. As seen in the occlusal view, the thickness of the tooth buccolingually masks the carious lesion when it is small **(Figs 13.1A and B)**.

The actual depth of penetration of a carious lesion is actually deeper than it appears on the radiograph.

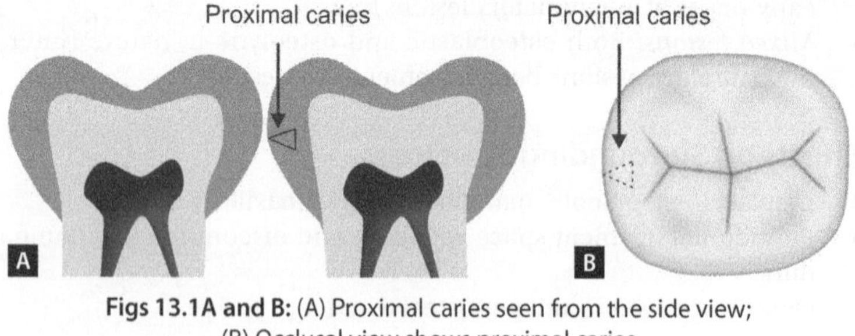

Figs 13.1A and B: (A) Proximal caries seen from the side view; (B) Occlusal view shows proximal caries

Factors Affecting Appearance of Caries on Radiographs

- *Buccolingual thickness of tooth:* The thicker the tooth, the more difficult it is to see the extent of the caries.
- *Limitations of two-dimensional film:* The extent of carious involvement cannot be seen in a buccolingual (cheek to tongue) direction.
- *X-ray beam angle (horizontal or vertical):* This is especially important when trying to identify recurrent caries, since changes in angulation may cause the superimposition of the existing restoration with the carious lesion. Overlap due to improper horizontal angulation makes it very difficult to diagnose early interproximal caries.
- *Exposure factors:* Caries detection is improved with a lower kVp setting, which provides a higher contrast. If the overall density of the film is too light or too dark, the diagnostic potential of the film is limited.

Transillumination

In the anterior region, interproximal caries can often be diagnosed using transillumination, which involves directing a bright light through the contact areas. Combining transillumination with radiographs enhances the diagnostic information obtained.

PROXIMAL CARIES

- Proximal caries commences apical (below) to the contact point.
- Starts off as a radiolucent *notch.*
- Later *cone-shaped* with the base toward the periphery.
- Sometimes-Hourglass shape contacting the dentin.
- At the D-E junction the caries spreads out forming a *another cone* shaped lesion with the *base toward the apex of the first cone.*
- The second cone appears to be mushrooms and then it is diffuse shaped.
- The outline of the caries is poorly demarcated.

Classification **(Figs 13.2 and 13.3)**

Incipient interproximal caries: Extends less than half way through the thickness of enamel. The term incipient means beginning to exist or appear. An incipient lesion, Class 1, is seen in enamel only.

Moderate interproximal caries: Extends more than halfway through the thickness of enamel but does not involve the dentinoenamel junction. A moderate lesion, Class 2, is seen in enamel only.

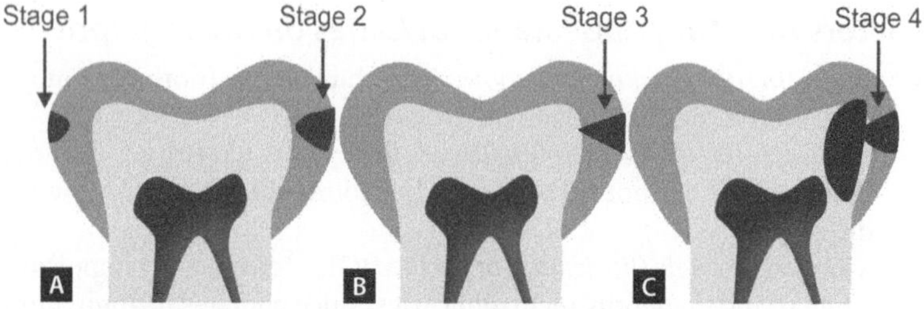

Figs 13.2A to C: Different stages of proximal dental caries. (A) *Stage 1:* Incipient, *Stage 2:* Moderate; (B) *Stage 3:* Advanced; (C) *Stage 4:* Severe

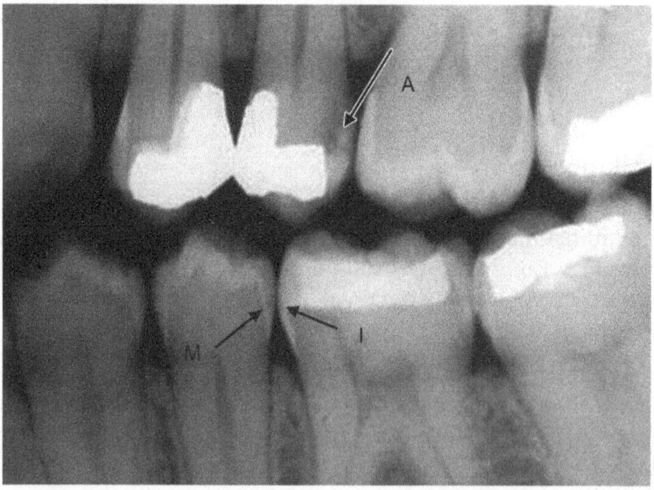

Fig. 13.3: Bitewing radiograph reveals incipient proximal carious lesion involving mesial surface of mandibular first molar (arrow, I), moderate caries on distal surface of second premolar (arrow, M) and advanced lesion on distal surface of second premolar (arrow, A)

Advanced interproximal caries: Extends to or through the dentino-enamel junction and into dentin but does not extend through the dentin more than half the distance toward the pulp. An advanced, Class 3, lesion affects both enamel and dentin.

Severe interproximal caries: Extends through enamel, through the dentin, and more than half the distance toward the pulp. A severe, Class 4, lesion involves both enamel and dentin and may appear clinically as a cavitation in the tooth.

OCCLUSAL CARIES

- It commences in pits and fissures. May occur at the base of a pit or fissure with no clinical signs.
- Not seen radiographically until the D-E junction reached.
- First seen as radiolucent dot at depth of fissure.
- Spreads out as thin radiolucent line at D-E junction.
- Later becomes conical with rounded apex *toward the pulp* and the base toward the periphery. Caries usually cannot be seen radiographically in the enamel.
- The caries first penetrates the dentin in a cone-shape with the base toward the periphery.
- The radiolucent outline is poorly demarcated.
- Outline later becomes diffuse.

Classification **(Figs 13.4A to D)**

Incipient occlusal caries: Cannot be seen on a dental radiograph and must be detected clinically with an explorer.

Moderate occlusal caries: Extends into dentin and appears as a very thin radiolucent line. The radiolucency is located under the enamel of the occlusal surface of the tooth. Little, if any radiographic change is noted on the enamel **(Fig. 13.5)**.

Severe occlusal caries: Extends into dentin and appears as a large radiolucency. The radiolucency extends under the enamel of the occlusal surface of the tooth. Severe occlusal caries is apparent clinically and appears as a cavitation in a tooth **(Fig. 13.5)**.

BUCCAL AND LINGUAL CARIES

It involves the buccal tooth surface, whereas lingual caries involves the lingual tooth surface. Because of the superimposition of the densities of normal tooth structure, buccal or lingual caries are difficult to detect on

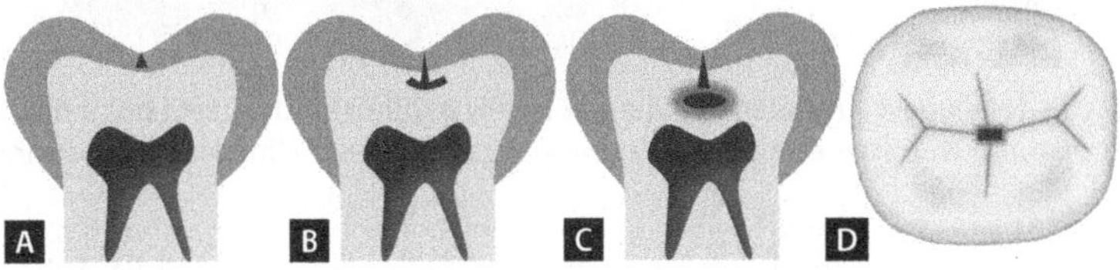

Figs 13.4A to D: Types of occlusal dental caries. (A) Incipient; (B) Moderate; (C) Advanced; (D) Occlusal caries starts as by deepening of occlusal pits and fissures

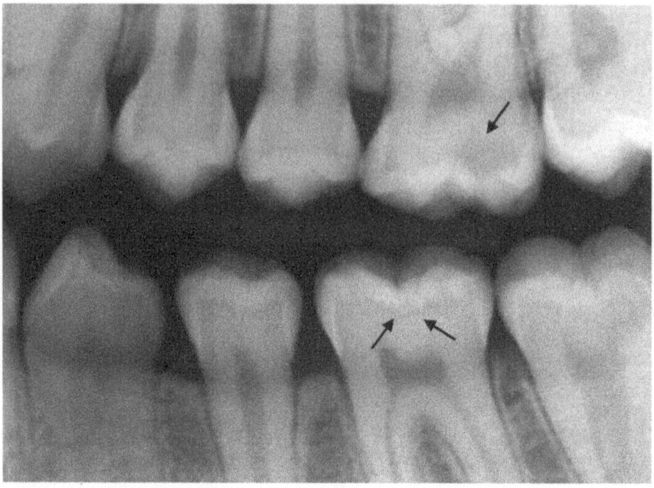

Fig. 13.5: Moderate occlusal caries seen on lower first molar (arrows) and severe occlusal caries (arrow) on upper first molar tooth

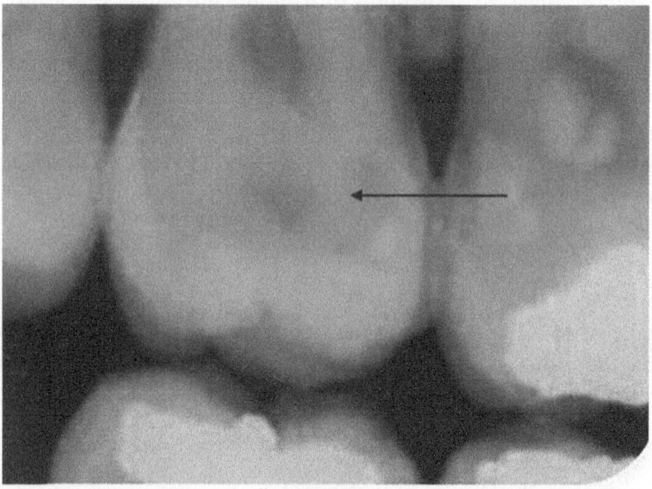

Fig. 13.6: Lingual caries seen as radiographically as diffuse radiolucent but difficult to distinguish between buccal and lingual caries unless clinical examinations

a dental radiograph and are best detected clinically **(Fig. 13.6)**. When viewed on a dental radiograph, caries that involves the buccal or lingual surface appears as a small, circular radiolucent area. To determine the location of the lesion, a clinical examination with an explorer is necessary.

ROOT SURFACE CARIES

Root caries involves only the roots of the teeth. The cementum and dentin located just below the cervical region of the tooth is involved and no involvement of enamel occurs. Bone loss and corresponding gingival recession precede the caries process and result in exposed root surfaces. Clinically, root surface caries is easily detected on exposed root surfaces. The most common locations include the exposed roots of the mandibular premolar and molar areas. On a dental radiograph, root surface caries appears as a cupped-out or crater-shaped radiolucency just below the cementoenamel junction (CEJ) **(Fig. 13.7)**. Early lesions may be difficult to detect on dental radiograph.

SECONDARY OR RECURRENT CARIES

Recurrent caries occurs adjacent to a pre-existing restoration. On a dental radiograph, recurrent caries appears as a radiolucent area just beneath a restoration. Recurrent caries occurs most often beneath the interproximal margins of a restoration **(Fig. 13.8)**.

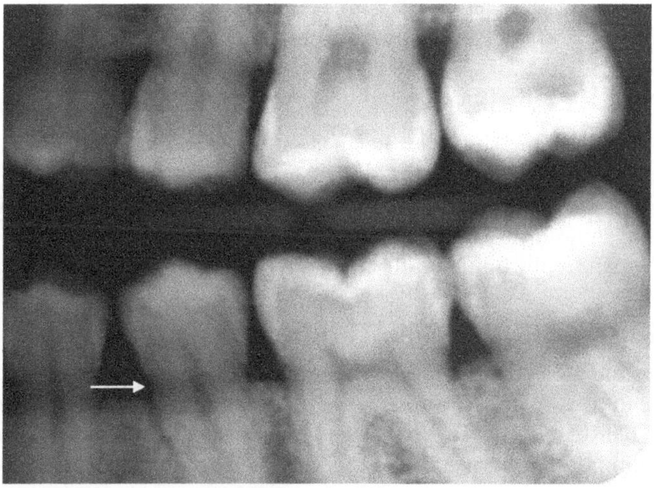

Fig. 13.7: Root surface caries appears as a crater-shaped radiolucency below the cementoenamel junction

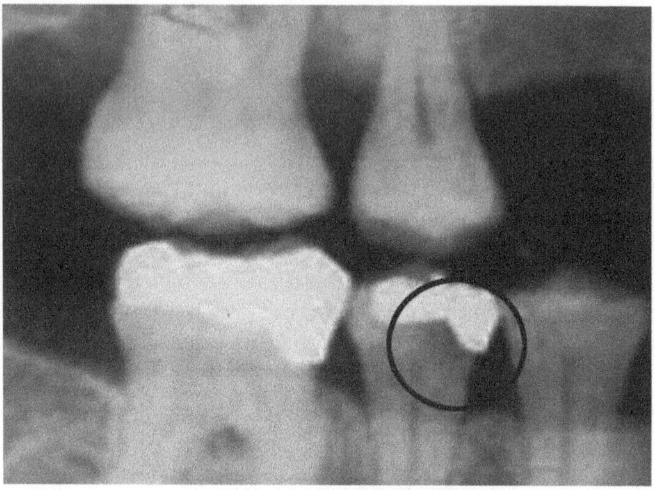

Fig. 13.8: Recurrent caries seen below the amalgam restoration on lower second premolar

ARRESTED CARIES

- Seen on proximal surface of tooth as a vague radiolucent notch where adjacent tooth is lost, i.e. no contact.
- Arrested caries in pits or fissures rarely seen.
- Can be mistaken for cervical burnout.

RAMPANT CARIES

- Usually occurs in children on high carbohydrate diet, poor oral hygiene and no fluorides.
- Seen radiographically as diffuse radiolucent areas. Interproximal and smooth surfaces affected.
- Nursing/baby bottle syndrome is a type of rampant caries.

RADIATION/DRUG-RELATED CARIES

- Found in head/neck radiation therapy patients with xerostomia.
- Due to xerostomia and not only the teeth in the beam affected. A type of rampant caries that usually is seen as a radiolucent shadow commencing at the necks (cervical caries) of teeth and spreads mesially and distally in patients with poor oral hygiene not using topical fluoride.

- Several adjacent teeth often affected causing crowns to be lost with root fragments remaining.
- Many patients are taking drugs that produce xerostomia and that can result in a similar appearance.

CERVICAL BURNOUT

Cervical burnout is an apparent radiolucency found just below the CE junction on the root due to anatomical variation (concave root formation posteriorly) or a gap between the enamel and bone covering the root (anteriorly) and mimics root caries. Posteriorly, this radiolucency usually disappears when another film of the region is examined. Caries does not occur on the root of the tooth unless there is loss of alveolar bone and gingival tissue due to recession or periodontitis.

Posterior Cervical Burnout

The invagination of the proximal root surfaces allow more X-rays to pass through this area, resulting in a more radiolucent appearance on the radiograph **(Fig. 13.9)**. X-rays directed at a different angle usually pass through more tooth structure and the radiolucency disappears **(Figs 13.10A and B)**.

Anterior Cervical Burnout

The space between the enamel and the bone overlying the tooth will appear more radiolucent than either the enamel or the bone-tooth combination.

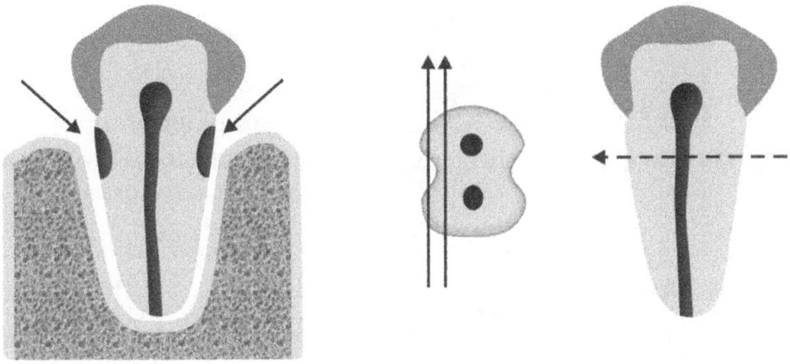

Fig. 13.9: Cervical burnout occurs due to convergence of tooth portions just below the cementoenamel junction allow more X-rays to pass through this area results in radiolucent at CE junction

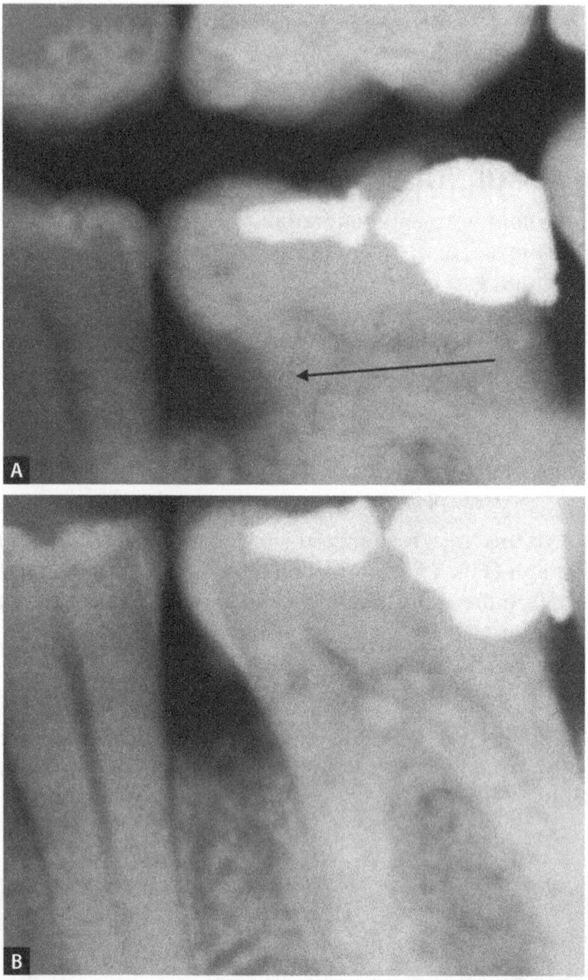

Figs 13.10A and B: (A) Cervical burnout appears on mesial surface of lower first molar; (B) On periapical projection, cervical burnout disappears

MACH BAND EFFECT

Optical illusion giving appearance of increased radiolucency at the junction of differing tissue densities, such as enamel and dentin. If you block off the enamel with a fingernail, the radiolucency will disappear, if due to the Machband effect. If the radiolucency persists, it may be caries.

EFFECTIVENESS OF RADIOGRAPHS IN THE DETECTION AND EVALUATION OF DENTAL CARIES

To increase the effectiveness of radiographs in the detection of dental caries, care must be given to ensure that:

- The common radiographic technique errors are avoided, such as ensuring that the bitewing film used to detect dental caries must be free of overlapped contacts and that the horizontal angulation is proper, so that overlapping of the contact areas of the crowns of the teeth is avoided.
- Technique variations in film and X-ray beam positions can considerably affect the image of the carious lesion. For example, varying the horizontal angulation can make a lesion confined to enamel appear to have progressed into dentine. Hence, there is the need for accurate, reproducible techniques.
- Radiographic diagnosis of caries is also limited by problems such as that carious lesions are always larger clinically than they appear radiographically and very early lesions are often not evident at all.
- A number of radiolucencies that involve the crowns and the roots of teeth often seen on a dental radiograph and may be confused with dental caries.
- Radiolucent restorative materials, abrasion, attrition and cervical burnout may all resemble dental caries on a radiograph. Hence, the final diagnosis of caries should only be made after the clinical and radiographic findings are corroborated. Both the clinical examination and the interpretation of radiographs are mutually contributory aids in making the diagnosis of dental caries.

CHAPTER 14

Radiographic Interpretation of Periodontal Diseases

Clinical examination in establishing the diagnosis and guiding the treatment plan for a patient affected by those periodontal diseases which have contributed to destruction of the periodontal attachment. A range of findings of relevance to clinically evident periodontal conditions can become apparent on radiographs. Radiographs can provide key information of relevance to periodontal decision making which is not capable of being captured by clinical examination, such as length of root with remaining bony support.

The role of radiographs offering information in the diagnosis of periodontal diseases and in guiding management of periodontal diseases at various stages of treatment.

VALUE OF PERIODONTAL RADIOGRAPHY

Periodontal disease is the major health problem, and therefore appropriate diagnosis has become very important. The periodontium is the three-dimensional group of tissues, structures and substances which represent different level of X-ray beam penetration. A clinical evaluation of the periodontium (periodontal probing) is always performed first, followed by the radiographic study.

LIMITATIONS OF RADIOGRAPHY IN PERIODONTAL DISEASES

The major limitations of radiographic evaluation of the alveolar bone are:

- Dental radiographs will not show changes until more than 30–60% bone resorption have occurred.
- There are certain situations where clinical examination is necessary for proper diagnosis, for example, if the bone loss occurs on the lingual or buccal/palatal site of the alveolar bone only.
- The early stage of periodontal disease (gingivitis) is not radiographically evident, and therefore clinical evidence of disease precedes radiographic changes.

- The first grade of furcation involvement is not evident radiographically.
- Appropriate evaluation of the radiographs depends on the quality of exposure, which requires correct positioning and conditions. Under exposed, burnout and malpositioned radiographs are nondiagnostic.

RADIOGRAPHIC TECHNIQUES

To determine adequate angulation of periapical radiographs, there are four criteria:

1. The radiograph should show the tips of molar cusps with little or none of the occlusal surface showing.
2. Enamel and pulp chambers should be distinct.
3. Interproximal spaces should be open.
4. Proximal contacts should not overlap unless teeth are out of line anatomically.

Techniques

- The optimal projections for periodontal diagnosis in the posterior teeth are bitewing radiographs.
- If significant amounts of bone loss are suspected (based on clinically assessment including probing depths and gingival recession), vertical bitewing radiographs are indicated.
- In the anterior, anterior periapical projections, exposed using the paralleling technique, are adequate.
- Anterior bitewing projections are also used for assessing periodontal disease.
- Posterior periapical projections tend to display somewhat foreshortened views of the maxillary molar teeth. The foreshortening of the image tends to project the buccal plate of bone coronally. The resultant image displays greater bone height than actually exists.
- Exposure factors also play a role in increasing the diagnostic yield from the radiographs.
- By using a higher kVp setting (90 kVp), instead of the customary 70 kVp, and reducing the mAs, a radiograph with a wider gray scale will be produced. This allows subtle changes in bone density, as well as soft tissue outlines, to be discerned.
- The X-ray beam must be perpendicular to the long axes of the teeth and the plane of the image receptor. The image receptor must be parallel to the long axes of the teeth.

To evaluate periodontal diseases different radiographic views are needed. It is also mentioned that radiographs produced with the bisecting angle technique may appear to indicate greater destruction of the alveolar bone than is actually present.

NORMAL APPEARANCE OF PERIODONTAL TISSUES (FIG. 14.1)

The periodontal hard tissues consist of cementum and alveolar bone. The radiographic appearance of healthy human periodontal tissues is as follows:

- The bone height is within 2 mm of the cementoenamel junction (CEJ).
- The crestal bone is a continuation of the lamina dura of the teeth, and is continuous from tooth to tooth.
- Between the anterior teeth, the alveolar crest is pointed.
- Between the posterior teeth, the lamina dura and the crestal bone form a box, with sharp angles.
- The periodontal ligament space varies along the length of the roots. It tends to be wider at the apex and alveolar crest and narrower in the midroot areas.
- The spongious bone appearance in the periapical area should be the same as in interalveolar region.

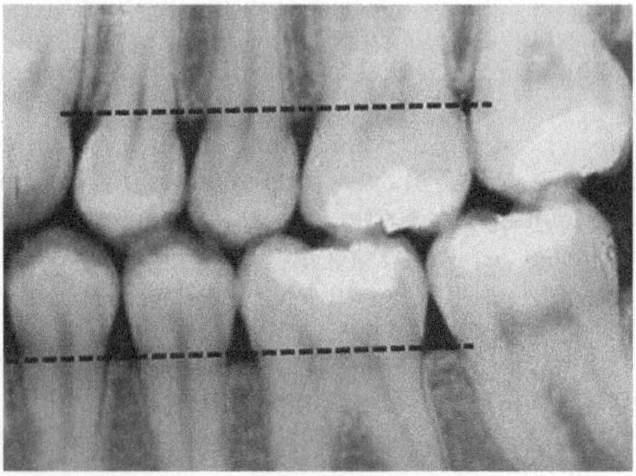

Fig. 14.1: Appearance of alveolar crest bone at the level of cementoenamel junction indicating healthy periodontium

Radiography in Periodontal Disease and Other Pathologic Conditions

Numerous mechanical, metabolic, inflammatory and microbiological factors influence the quality, density and structure of periodontal tissues, resulting in radiographic changes. Various periodontal diseases, which characterize the process of attachment destruction, bone loss, and other changes.

- *Lamina dura:* In early periodontitis, lamina dura visible as, continuous and linear but in advanced stage of periodontitis demonstrate, lamina dura loses its anatomic character.
- *The interalveolar septa* edges lose their sharpness; this is a very important sign of periodontal disease.
- *The periodontal ligament space* becomes widened and irregular in periodontal disease.
- *Vertical bone loss:* It occurs when there is one area of recession with the surrounding tissue being higher and closer to the CEJ.
  - *Early stage of bone loss:* Three wall bony pocket (surrounded by three bony walls); when both buccal and lingual cortical plates remain **(Fig. 14.2A)**.
  - Two wall defects described as, when one of these plates has been resorbed **(Fig. 14.2B)**.
  - One wall defect is, when both the buccal and lingual plates have been lost.
  - A four wall or circumferential defect occurs when the bone loss surrounds the entire tooth.

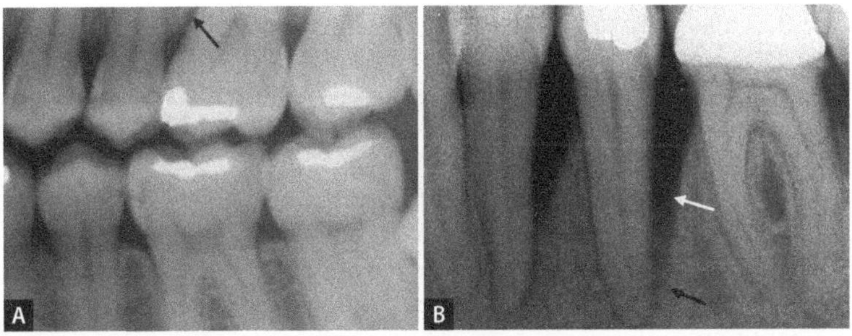

Figs 14.2A and B: (A) Appearance of early stage of bone loss in mild chronic periodontitis (arrow); (B) Advanced periodontitis shows severe bone loss up to the apex of the root; note lingual cortical plate is retained (white arrow) but buccal cortical plate is resorbed till apical end of the root (black arrow)

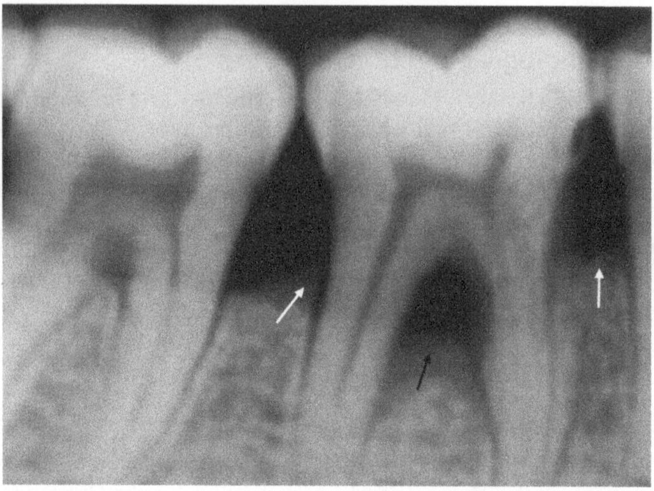

Fig. 14.3: Vertical bone loss seen in relation to distal aspect of first molar (white arrow) and grade 3 furcation involvement (black arrow) and horizontal on mesial aspect of the tooth (white arrow)

- *Furcation involvement:* Appears as a loss of density and lack of substance at the coronal aspect of the inter-radicular bone. Clinically, it has three grades:
  1. Grade 0—has no furcation involvement.
  2. Grade 1—the periodontal probe may be inserted into the furcation area but the destruction is less than one-third of the horizontal width.
  3. Grade 2—the probe explores the furcation but does not pass it through.
  4. Grade 3—total involvement; the probe passes through the furcation from one side to another of the multirooted teeth **(Fig. 14.3)**.
- *Radiographic appearance of calculus:* Visible subgingival deposits and tartar bridges joining adjacent teeth. Because calculus is radio-dense, in order to avoid interference of dental deposits on the final image, it is better to go for radiography after cleaned and scaled dentition.
- *Horizontal bone loss* is defined as an osteolytic process leading to a decreased height of the alveolar ridge and root exposure **(Fig. 14.4)**.
- *Ankylosis of the periodontal attachment* appears as the lack of a PDL space. The alveolar bone and root substance have no significant

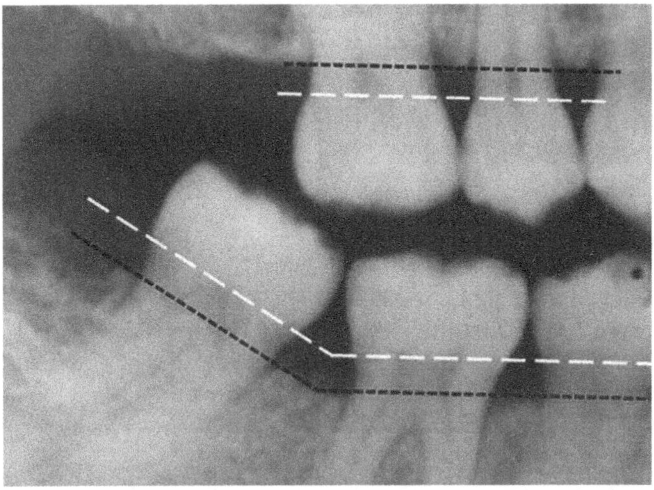

Fig. 14.4: Horizontal type of bone loss depicted as black dotted line and white dotted line indicates the level of alveolar crest in healthy periodontium on radiograph

borderline. Resorption of cementum is often followed by bone replacement of resorbed tissue.

- *Tooth luxation due to periodontal disease:* The tooth is pushed out from the alveolus due to loss of periodontal attachment. This is a long-term and atypical process. Usually, the tooth becomes loose (mobile).
- *Endoperiodontal lesions* (Class I) have primarily endodontic with subsequent periodontal involvement. Quite often, Class I lesions have fistulation. To distinguish the origin of the fistula, expose the radiograph after inserting a gutta percha point into intraoral opening.
- Radiograph of a "swimming tooth" with complete loss of periodontal attachment and level III mobility. High mobility of the tooth can be caused by loss of attachment as well as root fracture or neoplastic process. Radiographic assessment is necessary for diagnosis.

CHAPTER 15

Infection and Inflammation of the Jaws

Inflammatory lesions are the most common pathologic condition of the jaws. The source of infection and inflammatory agents, which causes periapical inflammatory lesions of the jaws are invading by means of deep dental caries, trauma to the teeth and periodontal disease.

When the infection spreads through the necrotic pulp tissues and restricted with in the apical region of the tooth called periapical infections. If it spreads through the bone marrow causing extensive lesions termed as osteomyelitis **(Flow chart 15.1)**.

PERIAPICAL INFECTIONS

Any evidence of radiological changes (i.e. radiolucent or radiopaque marks) suggests that there is some pathology of chronic stage, because in acute diseases, time is too short for any changes in the hard tissue that can be evident on the radiographical image **(Table 15.1)**.

Apical Periodontitis

It is the sequelae of pulp pathology where source of infection spreads through the deep dental caries involving pulpal tissue. Clinically,

Flow chart 15.1: Sequelae of pulpal pathology

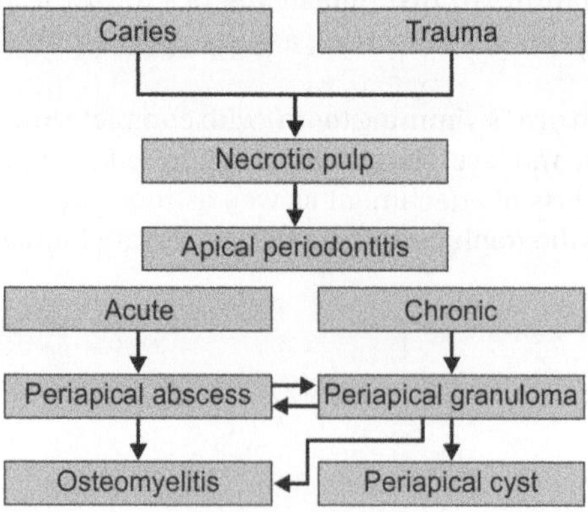

Table 15.1: Summary of the effects of different inflammatory processes on the periapical tissues and the resultant radiographic appearances

Stages of inflammation	*Underlying inflammatory changes*	*Radiographic appearances*
Initial acute inflammation	Inflammatory exudate accumulates in the apical periodontal ligament space (swelling) The tooth becomes tender to pressure (pain)	Widening of the radiolucent line of the periodontal ligament space or No apparent changes evident
Initial spread of inflammation	Resorption and destruction of the apical bony socket	Loss of the radiopaque line of the lamina dura at the apex
Further spread of inflammation	Further resorption and destruction of the apical alveolar bone	Area of bone loss at the tooth apex
Initial low-grade chronic inflammation	Minimal destruction of the apical bone. The body's defense systems lay down dense bone in the apical region	No apparent bone destruction but dense sclerotic bone evident around the tooth apex (sclerosing osteitis)
Latter stages of chronic Inflammation	Apical bone is resorbed and destroyed. The body's defense systems try to lay down dense bone around the area of resorption (Both processes are happening together)	Circumscribes, well-defined radiolucent area of bone loss at the apex, surrounded by dense sclerotic bone (periapical granuloma or cyst)

it presents as a nonvital tooth, and tooth is very sensitive to pressure and percussion. Pain is of throbbing type with regional lymph node enlargement.

Radiographic appearance: Initial stages show slight widening of periodontal ligament space in the apex of the tooth caused by edema with accumulation of inflammatory exudate in the periodontal ligament space. In advanced stages, loss of lamina dura in the apex **(Fig. 15.1B and C, Fig. 15.2)**.

Periapical Abscess

In acute periapical abscess, inflammatory response may extend to adjacent periapical alveolar bone causing necrosis of periapical tissues and diffuse rarefaction of bone leading to the formation of periapical abscess. The extent and degree of intensity of the pathology depends

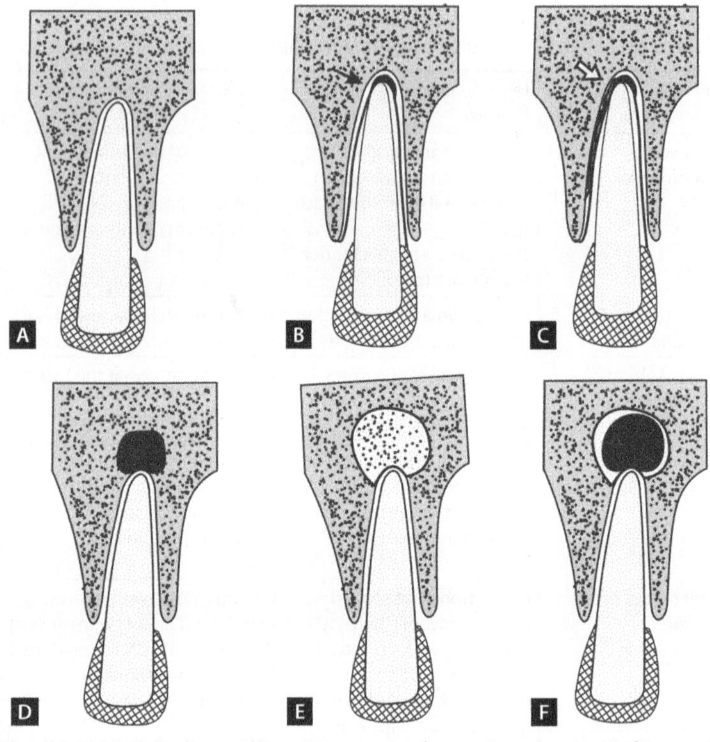

Figs 15.1A to F: Radiographic appearances of sequelae of pulpal inflammation. (A) Normal tooth; (B) Early periapical changes—widening of the periodontal space; (C) Loss of lamina dura; (D) Extensive acute inflammation—diffuse, ill-defined radiolucency in the apex; (E) Low-grade chronic inflammation—diffuse radiopaque area at the apex; (F) Long-standing chronic inflammation—well-defined radiolucency with sclerotic border

on the defensive mechanism of the body and the virulence of the microorganism.

Clinically, patient experiences severe pain with sensitive to pressure and percussion. Inflammatory exudate may spread along the tissue spaces results in the intra- or extraoral swelling.

Radiographically, acute periapical abscess shows, no changes occurs except there is widening of the periodontal ligament space, and some times, there is discontinuity of the lamina dura in the apical region. Chronic periapical abscess revealed that presence of round or oval radiolucency with ill-defined borders in the apex of the involved

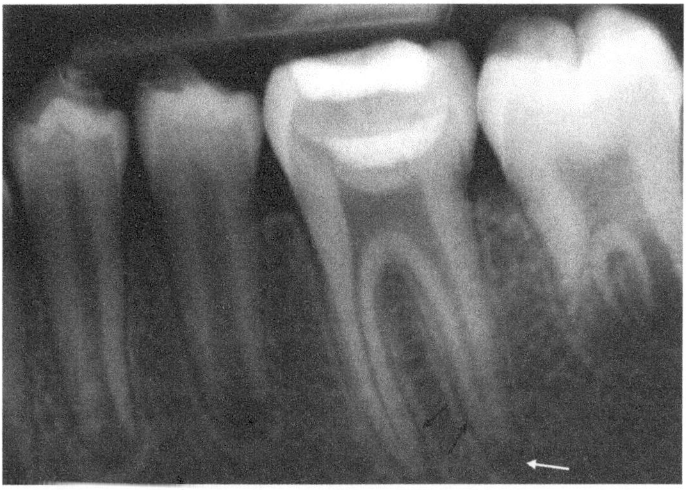

Fig. 15.2: Periapical radiograph shows widening of periodontal ligament space (black arrows) and loss of lamina dura at the apex of the distal root (white arrow)

tooth, complete or partial radiolucency depends upon the degree of bone loss **(Figs 15.3A and B, Fig. 15.1D)**.

Periapical Granuloma

Periapical granuloma is a localized mass of chronically inflamed granulation tissue at the apex of a nonvital tooth. The periapical granuloma results from pulpal death and necrosis, and is the most common sequelae of pulpal pathology. A periapical granuloma may give rise to a periapical cyst or periapical abscess. Clinically, it presents as a asymptomatic lesion unless, it get secondarily infected.

Radiographically, this appears as a widening of periodontal ligament space, loss of lamina dura in the apex of the tooth and presence of well-defined radiolucency at the apex. But it is differentiated from abscess by the well-defined with corticated borders **(Fig. 15.4, Figs 15.1E and F)**.

Periapical Cyst or Radicular Cyst

Periapical cyst results due to chronic irritation from the infected root canal lead to formation of granuloma which subsequent cystic degeneration. The epithelial lining of the cyst develops from the rests of Malassez in the periodontal ligament, which are stimulated to proliferate by inflammatory substances.

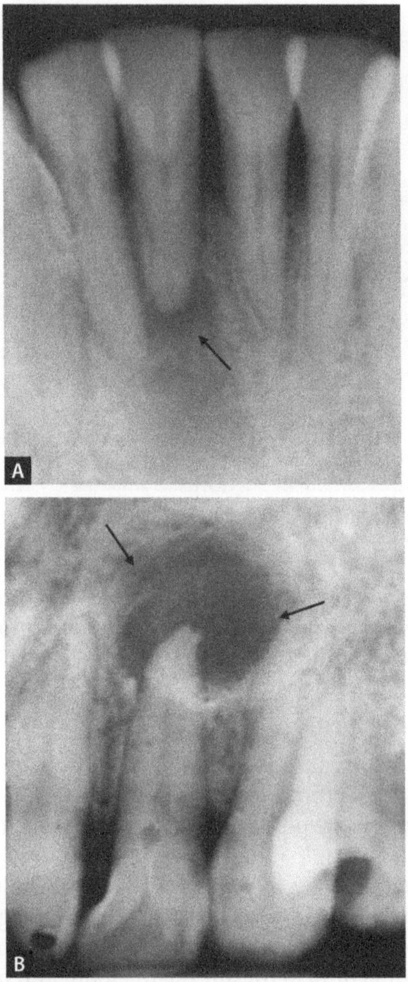

Figs 15.3A and B: (A) Early stage of chronic periapical abscess shows widening of periodontal ligament space, loss of lamina dura with small radiolucency with irregular margin at the apex of the root (arrow); (B) In advanced stage, large radiolucency with indistinct border (arrows)

Radicular cyst is the most common odontogenic cyst, represents an asymptomatic case clinically unless it may get infected.

Radiographically, it appears as a round or pear-shaped radiolucency at the apex of the non-vital tooth. There are no much differences

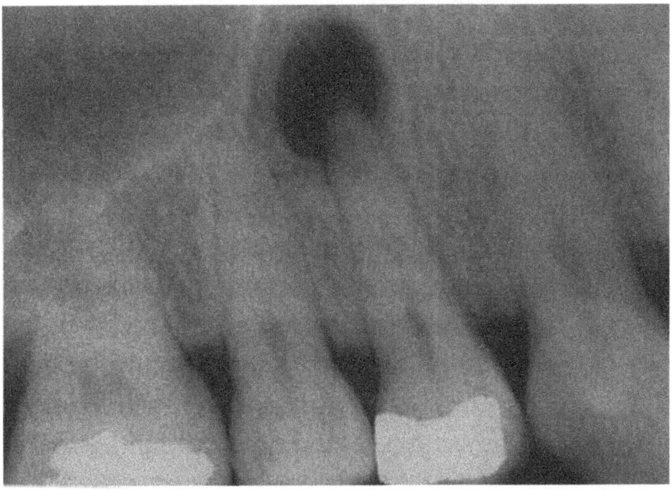

Fig. 15.4: Periapical granuloma on periapical radiograph; presents widening of periodontal ligament space, loss of lamina dura with well-demarcated radiolucency at the apex of the root. Note well-defined radiolucency with sclerotic border

between granuloma and cyst, if the radiolucency is more than 1.5 cm in diameter, the lesion is more likely a cyst, and the lesion is covered by thin radiopaque or sclerotic border, which is continuous with the lamina dura. In case of infected cyst, lesion shows loss of well-defined with sclerotic border **(Figs 15.1E and F, Fig. 15.5)**.

Pericoronitis

Inflammation of the pericoronal flap associated with the erupting or impacted tooth called as pericoronitis. The radiologic signs of pericoronitis can range from no changes, when the inflammatory lesion is confined to the soft tissues, to localized rarefication and sclerosis to osteomyelitis in the most severe cases.

An area of bone loss or radiolucency immediately distal to the crown of the impacted tooth. In extensive cases of pericoronitis, effects on surrounding structures as evidence of periosteal new bone formation at the inferior border of the mandible.

Osteomyelitis

Osteomyelitis is an inflammation of bone and bone marrow spaces. Osteomyelitis usually caused by pyogenic organisms that reach the

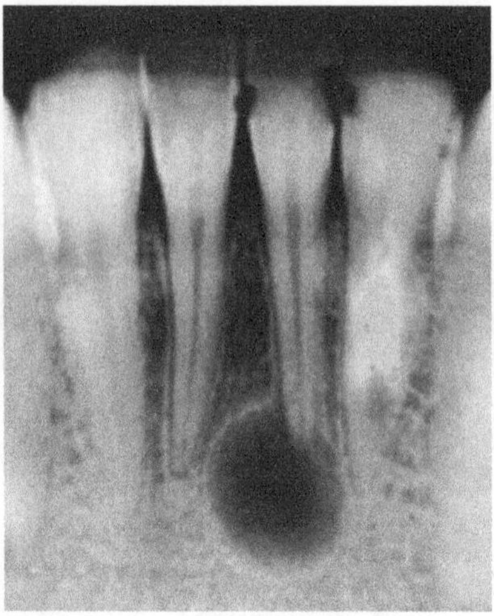

Fig. 15.5: Periapical radiograph revealed periapical cyst; widening of periodontal ligament space, loss of lamina dura and well demarcated with sclerotic (corticated) border radiolucency at the apex of the root

bone marrow from abscessed teeth or postsurgical infection, sometimes source of infection through the hematogenous spread.

Numerous forms of osteomyelitis have been described for the sake of simplicity; we group them into two major phases acute and chronic.

Acute Phase of Osteomyelitis

- The first radiographic evidence of the acute form of osteomyelitis is a slight decrease in the density of the involved bone with blurring of bony trabeculae.
- Bone destruction is more profound, resulting in an area of radiolucency in one focal area or in scattered regions through the involved bone.
- Later appearance of sclerotic regions becomes apparent.
- Sequestra may be present but usually more apparent and numerous in chronic form.
- Inflammatory exudate can lift the periosteum and stimulate bone formation. Radiographically, this appears as a thin, faint, radiopaque line adjacent to the surface of the bone. As lesion develops more number of new bone layer forms parallel to each other appears as an *Onion-skin*.

Chronic Phase of Osteomyelitis

- Most of the lesion appeared as a more radiopaque or sclerotic bone pattern.
- Evidence of small radiopaque sequestra (small pieces of necrotic bone) within the area of bone destruction appeared as a *moth eaten.*
- Evidence of involucrum surroundings the area of destruction following extensive subperiosteal bone formation **(Fig. 15.6)**.

Condensing Osteitis or Chronic Focal Sclerosing Osteomyelitis

It is a mild chronic inflammation which irritates the periapical tissue to form sclerotic changes. The source of infection through the pulpal pathology.

Radiographically, this appears as a **(Fig. 15.7)**:

- Loss of lamina dura in the periapical portion.
- Widening of periodontal ligament space.
- Radiopaque lesion or sclerotic bone occurs in the periapical area.

Condensing osteitis usually confused with fibro-osseous lesions where a radiopaque lesion does not contact with the tooth and lesions

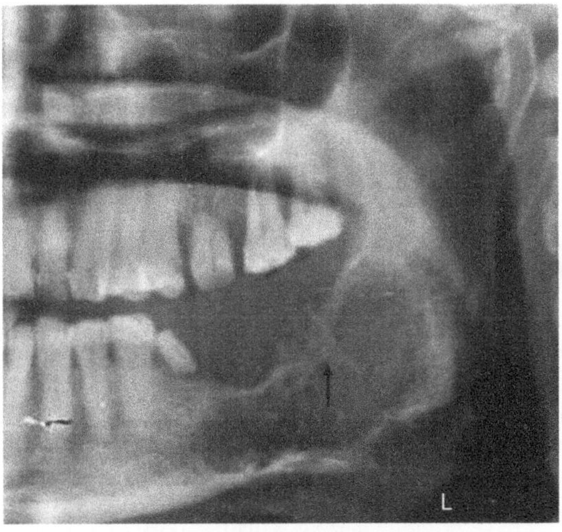

Fig. 15.6: Osteomyelitis of lower left jaw. Cropped panoramic shows extensive destruction of bone appears as "moth-eaten". Note radiopaque structure (sequestrum) surrounded by radiolucent and new bone formation (involucrum) at the periphery of the lesion (arrow)

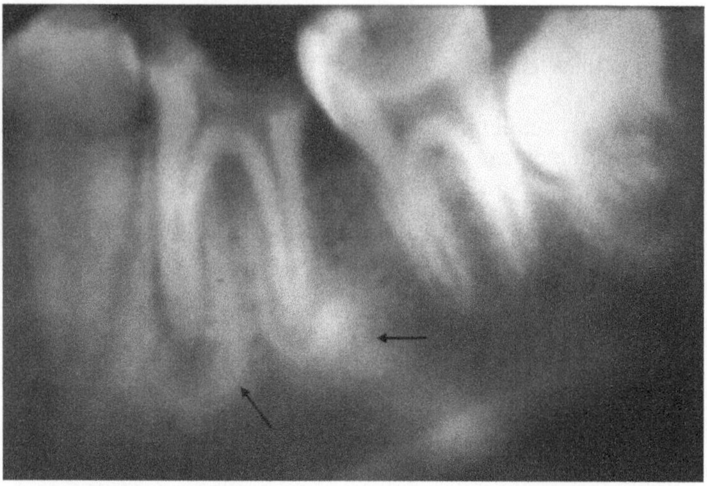

Fig. 15.7: Chronic focal sclerosing osteomyelitis of periapical radiograph depicting radiopaque lesions at both the root apex (arrows)

are associated with the vital tooth without loss of lamina dura or widening of periodontal ligament space.

Osteoradionecrosis

Osteoradionecrosis refers to an inflammatory condition of bone (osteomyelitis) that occurs between 3 months to 4 years after the bone exposed to therapeutic radiation.

Osteoradionecrosis occurs when the therapeutic radiation dose is given above 50 Gy.

Etiology (Flow chart 15.2)

Predisposing factors which causes osteoradionecrosis are:
- Radiation
- Infection
- Poor oral hygiene
- Hypovascularity of bone
- Hypoxia of bone
- Hypocellularity of bone.

The three-stage classification proposed by Marx and Myers:
- *Stage* 1: Less than 2 mm of exposed bone with or without pain and with radiological signs of diffuse demineralization;

Flow chart 15.2: Pathophysiology of osteoradionecrosis

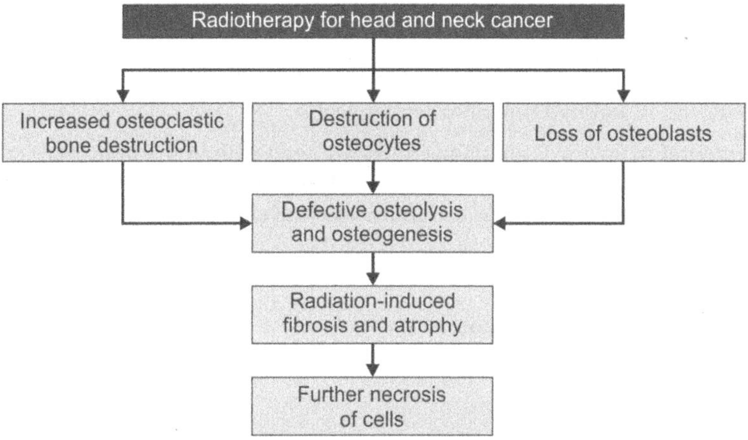

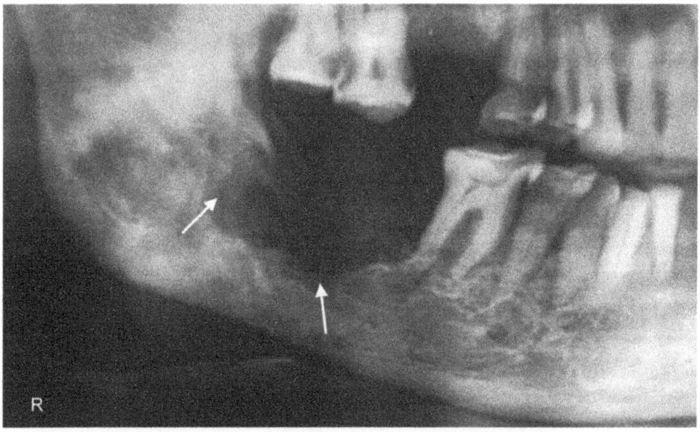

Fig. 15.8: Osteoradionecrosis. Extensive bone loss with new bone formation appears as mixed radiopaque and lucent lesions (arrows)

- *Stage* 2*:* More than 2 mm of exposed bone;
- *Stage* 3*:* Pathological fracture, oral fistula, fistula or lesion of the inferior border of the mandible. Clinically, it involved mandible more frequently than maxilla because of less vasculature and micro-anatomy of mandible.

Dental extraction or oral ulceration during or after radiotherapy leads to loss of epithelial layer and exposure of bone result into necrosis due to loss of vascularity from the periosteum and subsequently sequestrates leading to exposure of more bone associated with the intense pain and swelling.

Site: Frequently, it involves the posterior part of mandible.

Outline: Ill-defined similar to osteomyelitis.

Internal structure: Radiopaque areas are seen with in the radiolucency because of more bone formation within the destructed bony areas appeared granular similar to chronic osteomyelitis **(Fig. 15.8)**.

Effects: Stimulation of new bone formation on the outer cortex.

Differential diagnosis:
- Squamous cell carcinoma
- Chronic osteomyelitis.

CHAPTER 16

Radiographic Features of Jaw Cysts

A cyst is a pathologic cavity filled with fluid, lined by epithelium, and surrounded by connective tissue wall. The cystic fluid either is secreted by the cells lining the cavity or derives from the surrounding tissue fluid.

Cysts occur more frequently in the jaws because most cysts originate from the odontogenic epithelium. Cysts are radiolucent lesions, clinically they represents as a painless swelling and missing teeth.

Cysts are mainly grouped into two types:

1. *Odontogenic cysts:* Cysts are derived from the odontogenic epithelium.
2. *Nonodontogenic cysts:* Derived other than odontogenic epithelium.

CLASSIFICATION

1. *Odontogenic cysts:*
   - Radicular cyst
   - Dentigerous cyst
   - Residual cyst
   - Odontogenic keratocyst (Primordial cyst)
   - Basal cell nevus syndrome
   - Lateral periodontal cyst
   - Gingival cyst of the adult
   - Globulomaxillary cyst
   - Median mandibular cyst
   - Calcifying epithelial odontogenic cyst (Gorlin cyst)

- *Nonodontogenic cysts:*
  - Nasopalatine cyst
  - Median palatine cyst
  - Nasoalveolar cyst
  - Dermoid cyst
- *Pseudocysts:*
  - Simple bone cyst (traumatic bone cyst)
  - Aneurysmal bone cyst
  - Mucous retention cyst
  - Stafne's bone cyst

ODONTOGENIC CYSTS

Dentigerous Cyst (Follicular Cyst)

Dentigerous cyst is a cyst that forms around the crown of an unerupted tooth. It develops when fluid accumulates in the layers of reduced enamel epithelium or between the epithelium and the crown of the unerupted tooth **(Fig. 16.1)**.

Dentigerous cyst are the most common cyst after the radicular cyst in the jaws. Dentigerous cyst usually found in the mandibular third molar or the maxillary canine region because these teeth are most commonly impacted.

Age: Usually adolescents or young adults, 20–40 years.

Site: Mandibular third molar region and maxillary canine region.

Size: Variable, cyst suspected when follicular space exceeds 3 mm, but may grow several centimeters in diameter.

Shape:
- Round or oval typically envelops the crown symmetrically.
- Unilocular.

Outline:
- Smooth
- Well-defined
- Well-corticated

Internal structure: Completely radiolucent except for the crown of the involved tooth.

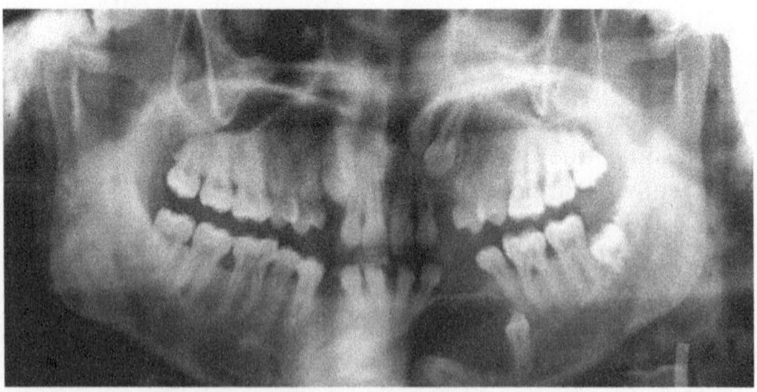

Fig. 16.1: Orthopantomograph revealed dentigerous cyst extending from the lower left 2nd premolar to the right canine region involving left lower canine, 1st premolar and right canine tooth

Effects:
- Associated tooth unerupted and displaced to apical direction
- Adjacent teeth are displaced and occasionally resorption occurs.
- Expansion of the medial or lingual cortical plate in such a extension causing facial asymmetry and displacement of the antrum.

Odontogenic Keratocyst

It is a noninflammatory odontogenic cyst that arises from the dental lamina. The epithelial lining of cyst is keratinized, hence the name as keratocyst.

High recurrence: The recurrence rate of odontogenic keratocyst is very high, due to the following reasons:
- *Daughter/satellite cyst formation:* Occasionally buds like proliferation of epithelium grow from the basal layer into the adjacent connective tissue wall. Also islands in the epithelium may give rise to satellite microcysts which is responsible for high propensity to recurrence because of these small microcysts or fragments of epithelium left behind after surgical intervention.
- *Collagenase activity of the cyst*
- *Remnant of dental lamina rest at the cyst wall*
- *Prostaglandin induced bone resorption*
- *Increase mitotic activity*

Age: Variable, peak incidence 2nd and 3rd decades.

Frequency: Less than 5% of all odontogenic cysts.

Site:
- Posterior body/angle of the mandible extends into the ramus.
- Anterior maxilla in canine region.

Shape: Oval, extending along the body of the mandible anteroposteriorly. Unilocular or multilocular.

Outline:
- Smooth
- Well-defined
- Well-corticated

Internal structure:
- Uniformly radiolucent.
- In some cases presence of internal septa give rise to multilocular appearances **(Fig. 16.2)**.

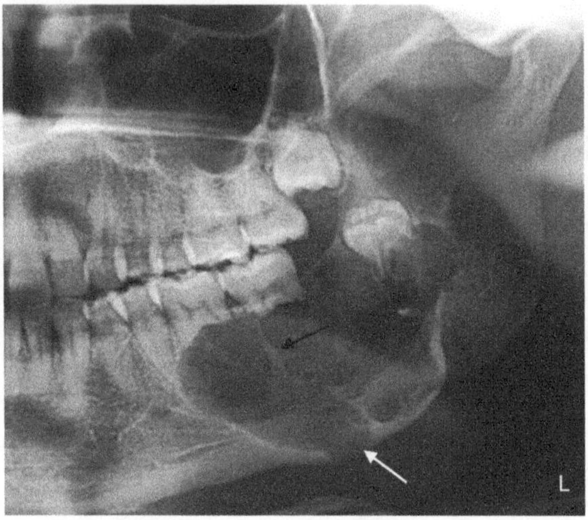

Fig. 16.2: Cropped panoramic image revealed odontogenic keratocyst; a multilocular well-corticated radiolucent with different septa (black arrow) and thinning of cortex (white arrow)

Effects:
- Minimal expansion of cortical plate because cyst extends anteroposteriorly rather than mediolaterally.
- Displacement and resorption of the tooth in a lesser extent than dentigerous cyst.
- Inferior alveolar canal displaced inferiorly.
- In maxilla cyst can invaginate and occupy the entire antrum.

Differential diagnosis:
- Dentigerous cyst
- Ameloblastoma
- Odontogenic myxoma
- Simple bone cyst.

Calcifying Epithelial Odontogenic Cyst (Gorlin Cyst)

It is an uncommon, slow growing, benign lesions. They occupy a spectrum ranging from a cyst to an odontogenic tumor. Now, it is categorized as a benign tumor.

Some instances lesion is associated with an odontoma. Clinically appears as a painless, slow growing located on either jaw anterior or premolar region.

Age: Peak age is 10–19 years of age.

Site: Equal distribution between the jaws. Most of the lesion occurs anterior to the first molar, especially cuspids and incisors.

Shape: Unilocular radiolucent lesion present in the bone.

Outline: Smooth, well-defined with corticated borders.

Internal structure: It appeared as a completely radiolucent lesion. In advanced stages small foci of calcified material appear as white flecks in the radiolucent area.

Effects:
- Displacement of teeth and resorption of roots may occur.
- Prevents the eruption of involved tooth.
- In larger lesions, perforates the cortical plate.

Residual Cyst

If cyst particularly radicular cyst not removed completely after extraction of involved tooth, remaining developed as residual cyst.

Residual cyst is asymptomatic and accidentally found during routine radiographic examination. Secondary infection of residual cyst can results in pain and expansion of bone.

Age: 5th decade

Site: Residual cyst occurs frequently in the mandible. It always located in the region where periapical cyst involved the tooth and commonly positioned above the inferior alveolar canal **(Fig. 16.3)**.

Shape: It appears as oval or circular in shape.

Outline: well-corticated border.

Internal structure: Residual cyst always shows solitary radiolucent lesion sometimes dystrophic calcification present in long standing case.

Effects: It can cause tooth displacement or resorption of root and buccal cortical plate expansion. It invaginated into the maxillary antrum or depresses the inferior alveolar canal.

Differential diagnosis: It can be diagnose only when the history or previous radiograph of periapical cyst.
- *Odontogenic keratocyst (OKC):* No cortical plate expansion since, it grows anteroposteriorly but residual cyst has a greater potential for bone expansion.
- *Stafne's cyst:* The epicenter always located below the inferior alveolar canal.

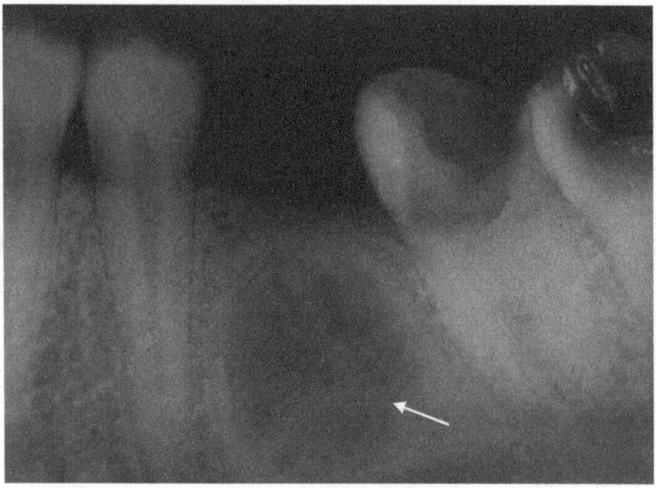

Fig. 16.3: Residual cyst; a well-defined corticated radiolucent at the extracted premolar area

Globulomaxillary Cyst

Globulomaxillary cyst is a fissural cyst of odontogenic in origin. It arises from the entrapment of epithelium during fusion of globular portion of medial nasal process with maxillary process in globulomaxillary suture. New concept say that, epithelium entrapment theory no longer accepted, however this cyst is now recognized as radicular cyst or lateral periodontal cysts or OKC.

Age: 2nd to 3rd decade.

Site: It located commonly between maxillary lateral incisor and canine.

Shape: It appears typically as a inverted pear shaped radiolucent with the apex pointed towards the alveolar crest between the roots of the maxillary lateral incisor and canine teeth.

Outline: Smooth corticated border.

Internal structure: Unilocular radiolucent lesion **(Fig. 16.4)**.

Effects: No symptom unless cyst becomes infected which causes pain and discomfort. Large cyst can cause buccal cortical bone expansion.

Differential diagnosis:

- *Lateral periodontal cyst:* Oval shaped radiolucency present
- *Lateral dentigerous cyst:* Associated with impacted tooth

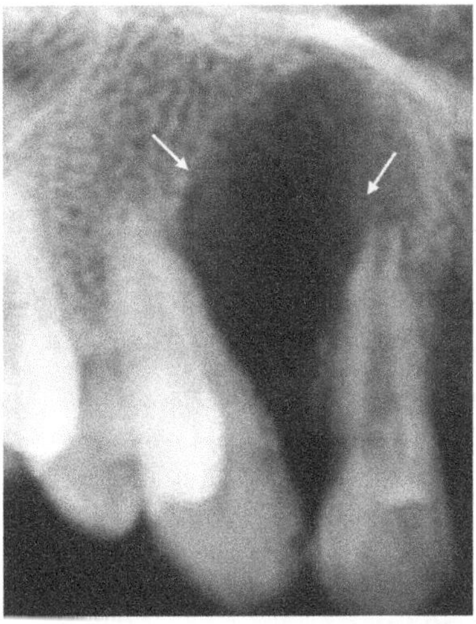

Fig. 16.4: Globulomaxillary cyst; note pear shaped radiolucency with apex towards the alveolar crest. Root resorption of maxillary lateral incisor with displacement of cuspid and lateral incisor

- *Adenomatoid odontogenic tumor:* Calcified flecks are visible within the lesion.
- *Traumatic bone cyst:* No fluid aspirated.
- *Gaint cell granuloma:* Anterior region

NONODONTOGENIC CYSTS

Nasopalatine Duct Cyst (Incisive Canal Cyst)

This cyst develops from epithelial remnants of the nasopalatine duct or incisive canal.

Age: Variable, but most frequently occurs in middle age (40–60 years of age).

Frequency: Accounts 10% of all jaw cysts.

Site: It occurs in nasopalatine foramen or incisive canal, located between the maxillary central incisors.

Shape:
- Round or oval
- Unilocular.

Outline:
- Smooth
- Well-defined
- Well-corticated (unless infected)

Internal structure: Uniformly radiolucent but radiopaque shadows sometimes superimposed.

Effects:
- Distal displacement of adjacent teeth and rarely resorbed.
- Palatal expansion.

Differential diagnosis:
- Large incisive foramen.
- Radicular cyst or periapical granuloma.

PSEUDOCYSTS

Aneurysmal Bone Cyst

Aneurysmal bone cyst is quite rare, benign, non-neoplastic, expansive, and vascular locally destructive lesions. It is generally considered sequelae of an earlier trauma causing an overflow of blood into the bone, though a number of pathogenic theories have been put forward. It is classified as pseudocysts because it exhibit no epithelial lining. It is an intraosseous accumulation of variable sized blood filled spaces surrounded by cellular fibrous connective tissue admixed with reactive woven bone.

Age: It is common among females before the age of 30 years.

Site: It is more common in mandible with an affinity towards molar and ramus region.

Shape: Oval or circular blow-out or ballooning distension of the normal contour of the affected bone.

Outline: well-defined border.

Internal structure: It is multilocular with wispy, ill-defined septa. These septa are positioned at right angles to the outer expanded border.

Effects: This cyst is extremely expansile. It can displace and resorb adjacent teeth. It may result in pain, paresthesia, crepitus, also mobility and migration of teeth leading to malocclusion. In maxillary cysts it can cause nasal obstruction, bleeding, proptosis and diplopia **(Fig. 16.5)**.

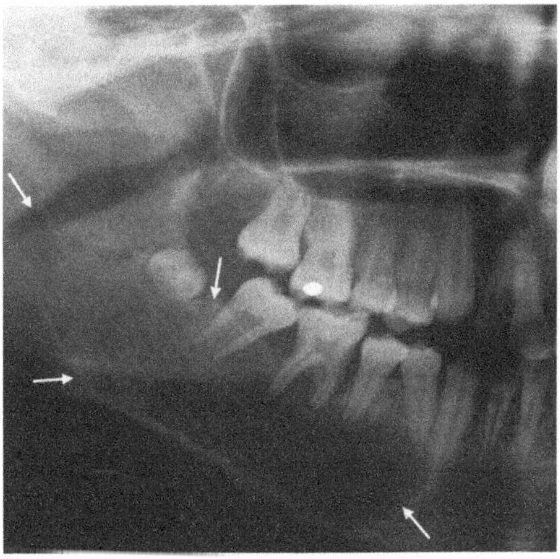

Fig. 16.5: Aneurysmal bone cyst, note thin septa within the radiolucent lesion appear as multilocular lesion with resorption of roots also observed

Differential diagnosis:
- *Ameloblastoma:* It also has a high tendency to cause expansion of cortical plate, but it is seen in older age group.
- *Central giant cell granuloma:* It results in similar radiographic appearance but its epicenter is located anterior to the first molar.
- *Central ossifying fibroma:* It appears as a mixed radiolucent-radio-opaque lesions.
- *Cherubism:* They have similar appearance but these occur bilaterally.

Traumatic Bone Cyst

It is not considered as a true cyst since it is not lined by epithelium. It has a connective tissue lining. It may or may not be associated with trauma. It has been noted that these cysts are found within the lesions of cemento-osseous dysplasia and fibrous dysplasia. This supports the fact that it is a localized error in normal bone remodelling or metabolism.

These are generally asymptomatic, become painful when the cyst is secondarily infected. There is seldom expansion of cortical plate and associated teeth are vital. These cysts are revealed on routine radiographic examination. On aspiration either a straw colored or serosanguinous fluid is evident. At times there may be no aspirate.

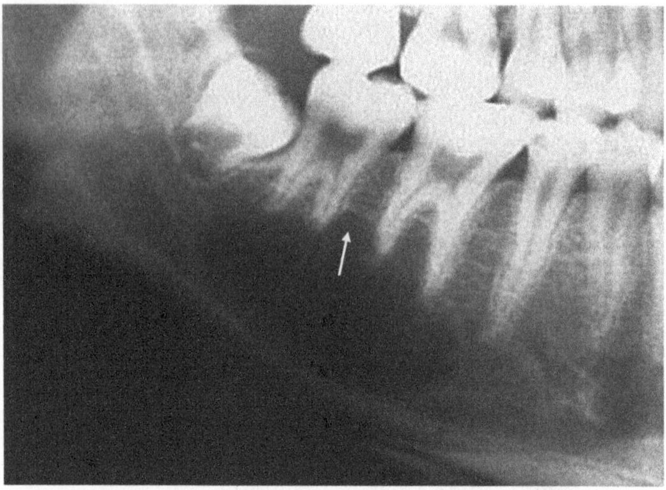

Fig. 16.6: Cropped panoramic radiograph shows a solitary large, ellipsoid, well-defined, corticated, lucent lesion; note scalloped border on superiorly (arrow)

Age: They are common in 1st and 2nd decades of life with slight male preponderance.

Site: These are common in posterior mandible and ramus area.

Shape: The cyst may be oval in shape.

Outline: These have variable margins ranging from a well-defined delicate cortex to ill-defined borders or have scalloped border. It scallops between the roots of the teeth **(Fig. 16.6)**.

Internal structure: It has a radiolucent internal structure or may give an illusion of multilocularity since there is scalloping in the endosteal surface of the cortical plates which superimpose on the cystic cavity.

Effects: This cyst has no influence on surrounding structures. It rarely causes root resorption or displacement of adjacent teeth. Even it spares the cortical boundary of the crypts around developing teeth.

Differential Diagnosis:

The dome like projections that scallop between the roots are highly suggestive of traumatic bone cyst. All the lesions which cause minimal expansion of bone are included in differential diagnosis.

- *Odontogenic keratocyst:* They have well-defined corticated borders and affect the adjacent teeth unlike traumatic bone cyst.
- *Radicular cyst:* As borders of traumatic bone cyst scallop between the roots, a radicular cyst should be ruled out. The teeth associated with traumatic bone cyst are vital.
- *Periapical cemento-osseous dysplasia:* The radiolucent stage can mimic it, but periapical cemento-osseous dysplasia is commonly seen in mandibular anteriors.

CHAPTER 17

Tumors of the Jaws

Tumors of the jaws **(Table 17.1)** generally divided into:

- *Benign:*

Odontogenic	*Nonodontogenic*
Ameloblastoma	Neurilemmoma
Adenomatoid odontogenic tumor	Neurofibroma
Calcifying epithelial odontogenic tumor	Neurofibromatosis
Odontoma	Osteoma
Ameloblastic fibro-odontoma	Central hemangioma
Ameloblastic fibroma	Arteriovenous fistula
Odontogenic myxoma	Osteoblastoma
Benign cementoblastoma	Chondroma

- *Malignant:*

Carcinoma	*Sarcoma*
Squamous cell carcinoma	Osteosarcoma
Primary intraosseous carcinoma	Chondrosarcoma
Mucoepidermoid carcinoma	Fibrosarcoma
Pleomorphic carcinoma	Ewing's sarcoma
Acinic cell carcinoma	Leukemia
Adenoid cystic carcinoma	Malignant lymphoma
Adenocarcinoma	Burkitt's lymphoma
	Multiple myeloma

BENIGN TUMORS OF THE JAWS

Benign tumors typically have an insidious onset and grow slowly. These are painless, do not metastasize and, not life-threatening unless they involved vital organ by direct extension. Benign tumors are detected clinically by swelling of the jaws and find a lesion radiographically.

Benign tumors of the jaws are classified into odontogenic (tumors arise from the odontogenic apparatus) and nonodontogenic (those arise from other than odontogenic tissues).

Table 17.1: Difference between radiographical general features of benign and malignant tumors

Benign tumor	*Malignant tumor*
Location: Odontogenic lesions occur naturally in the alveolar process above the inferior alveolar nerve canal where tooth formation occurs. Vascular and neural lesions may originate inside the mandibular canal arising from the neurovascular tissues. Cartilaginous tumors occur in jaws, where residual cartilage cells are present that is mandibular condyle.	**Location:** Primary and metastatic tumors occurs anywhere in the oral and maxillofacial region. Primary carcinomas occur commonly in the tongue, floor of the mouth, tonsils, lips, soft palate and gingiva and may invade the jaws from any of these sites. Sarcomas are common in mandible and posterior regions of both jaws. Metastatic tumors are common in posterior part of mandible and maxilla.
Periphery and shape: Typically have a smooth, round or oval periphery. Well-corticated and well-defined borders. Benign tumors are encapsulated, therefore show a radiolucent band separating the lesion from surrounding bone **(Figs 17.1A and B)**.	**Periphery and shape:** Malignant lesions are aggressively expanding outwards and cause erosion of the surrounding tissues. As a result of this the borders irregular, ragged and ill-defined. They have a mosaic form and blend with the normal tissue. Absence of encapsulation (absence of radiolucent outline) and cortication of borders **(Fig. 17.1C)**.
Internal structure: Benign tumors appeared as radiolucent, mixed and radiopaque lesions. Internal calcifications in the form of calcified flecks, septa are usually benign.	**Internal structure:** Which do not produce born or calcification, hence it appears only radiolucent.
Effects on surrounding structures: It exerts pressure on neighboring structures, resulting in the displacement of teeth and cortical bone expansion without discontinuity of periosteum and no perforation of bone or teeth. Root resorption occurs more in benign lesions (ameloblastoma, ossifying fibroma and central giant cell granuloma), but no resorption of root in fibro-osseous lesions **(Figs 17.2A and 17.3B)**.	**Effect on surrounding structure:** Rapid destruction of surrounding tissues causing floating teeth. Internal trabecular bone is destroyed and perforation of cortical bone occurs. No resorption or displacement of teeth **(Figs 17.2B and 17.3A)**.

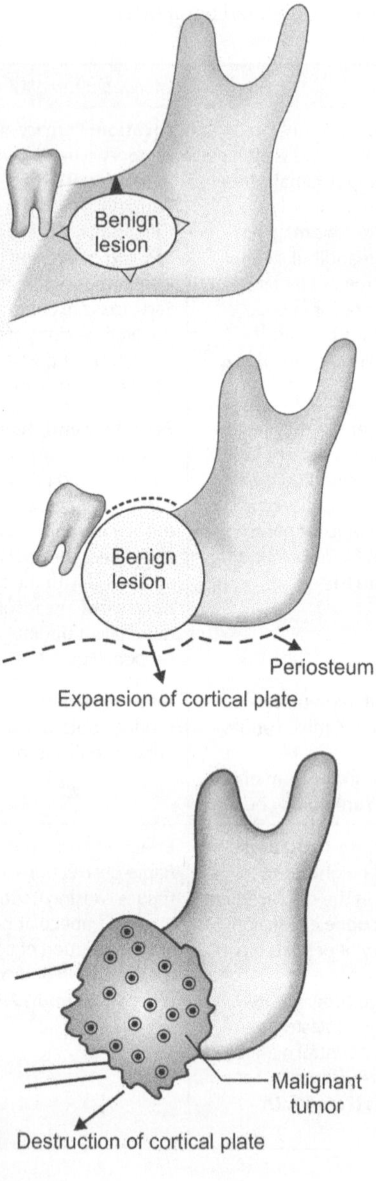

Figs 17.1A to C: (A and B) Benign lesions are growing by displacement and expansion of surrounding structures; (C) Malignant tumors are growing by invasion and destruction of surrounding bone without cortical expansion

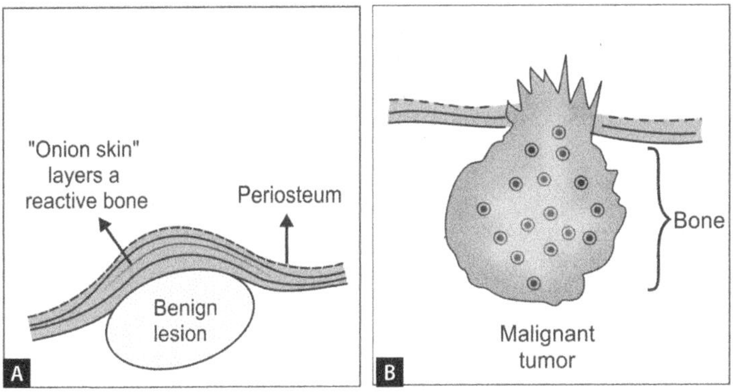

Figs 17.2A and B: (A) Benign lesions are growing near cortex cause expansion and formation of layers of reactive bone; (B) Malignant tumor growing near cortex cause destruction and rapid elevation of bone forming periosteum results in bony spicules resembling sunburst appearances

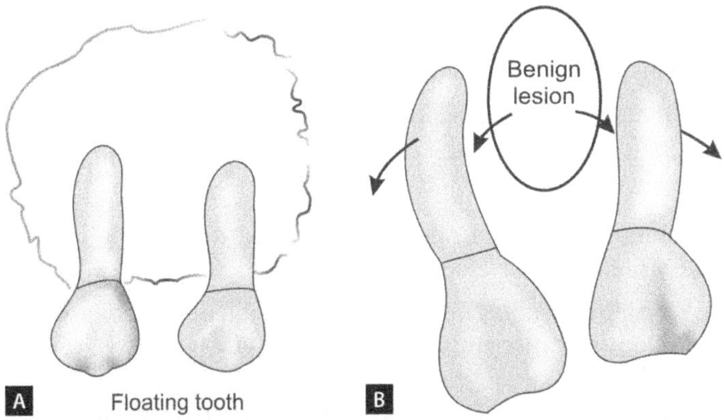

Figs 17.3A and B: (A) Malignant lesion spreads rapidly destroying bone but leaving teeth in position and without evidence of root resorption; (B) Benign lesion grows slowly, causing displacement and resorption of root

Odontogenic Tumors

Odontogenic tumors of the jaws are further classified into three groups:

1. Epithelial (ectoderm) odontogenic tumor
2. Connective tissue (mesoderm) odontogenic tumor
3. Mixed tissue (ecto- and mesoderm) odontogenic tumor.

Epithelial Odontogenic Tumors

- Ameloblastoma
- Calcifying epithelial odontogenic tumor
- Adenomatoid odontogenic tumor.

Mesodermal Odontogenic Tumors

- Odontogenic myxoma
- Odontogenic fibroma
- Cementoma.

Mixed Tissue

- Odontomas
- Ameloblastic fibroma
- Ameloblastic fibro-odontoma.

Ameloblastoma

Ameloblastoma is a true neoplasm of odontogenic epithelium of enamel organ or dental lamina. They are described as locally invasive but almost benign in its growth characteristics.

Age: Adults, about 40 years old.

Frequency: Rare, but still the most common odontogenic tumor.

Site:

- Posterior body/angle/ramus of mandible.
- Occasionally involves maxilla.

Size: Variable depending on the age of the lesion may become very large, if neglected and cause gross facial asymmetry.

Shape:

- In its early stage of development the ameloblastoma may appear as a unilocular radiolucency with no internal structure.
- Classical appearance is multilocular cystic like lesion with distinct septa dividing the lesion into large compartments of variable size appeared as *"soap bubble"* **(Fig. 17.4)** and numerous small compartments or loculations as a *"honeycomb appearance"* or *"tennis-racket pattern"*.

Outline:

- Smooth and scalloped
- Well-defined
- Well-corticated.

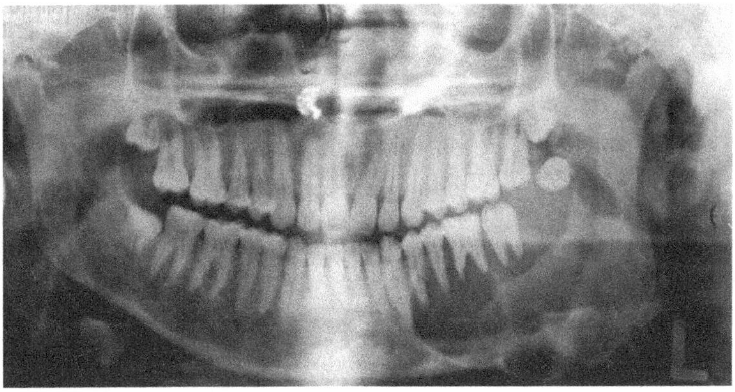

Fig. 17.4: Orthopantomogram (OPG) shows ameloblastoma with multilocular appearances on lower left angle of the mandible extends from left canine to ramus of the mandible on same side

Internal structure: Radiolucent with internal radiopaque septa.

Effects on surroundings structures:
- Extensive root resorption.
- Adjacent teeth displaced and loosened.
- Extensive expansion in all dimensions.
- Maxillary lesions can extend into the paranasal sinuses, orbit or base of the skull.

Differential diagnosis:
- Dentigerous cyst
- Radicular cyst
- Traumatic bone cyst
- Residual cyst
- Lateral periodontal cyst
- Giant cell granuloma.

Calcifying Epithelial Odontogenic (Pindborg) Tumor

It is a rare neoplasm of the tooth producing apparatus. They are located within the bone produce a mineralized substance of amyloid.

Age: Middle-aged adults.

Frequency: Very rare.

Site: Premolar/molar region of the mandible.

Size: 1–3 cm in diameter.

Shape:
- Usually unilocular often associated with unerupted tooth.
- Occasionally multilocular.

Periphery:
- Well-delineated (corticated)
- In some cases indistinct (diffuse) borders.

Internal structure: Mature lesion reveals a unilocular or multilocular cystic lesion with numerous scattered, radiopaque foci of varying size and density described as *driven snow appearance* **(Fig. 17.5)**.

Effects:
- Adjacent teeth sometimes displaced
- Resorption of involved tooth
- Prevent the eruption of tooth.

Differential diagnosis:
- Dentigerous cyst
- Ameloblastoma
- Central odontogenic fibroma
- Calcifying odontogenic cysts
- Odontoma (intermediate stage)
- Adenomatoid odontogenic tumors.

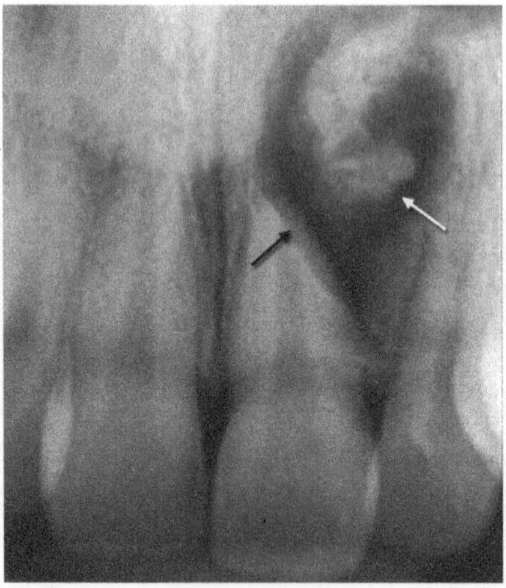

Fig. 17.5: Periapical radiograph showing calcifying epithelial odontogenic tumor with foci of calcification appears as driven snow (white arrow) and also resorption of root seen (black arrow)

Adenomatoid Odontogenic Tumor

Adenomatoid odontogenic tumors are uncommon, nonaggressive tumors of odontogenic epithelium.

Age: 5–50 years with average age is 16 years of female predilection.

Frequency: Rare tumor.

Site: 75% occurs in incisor-canine-premolar region of maxilla, rarely in mandible.

Shape: Unilocular radiolucency.

Outline:
- Well-defined
- Corticated or sclerotic border.

Internal structure:
- Variable
- Radiolucent lesion with foci of radiopaque **(Fig. 17.6)**.
- In some cases, lesion shows complete radiolucent.

Effects:
- Displaced adjacent teeth
- Root resorption is rare
- Inhibit eruption of involved tooth
- Expansion of jaw may occur but outer cortex maintained.

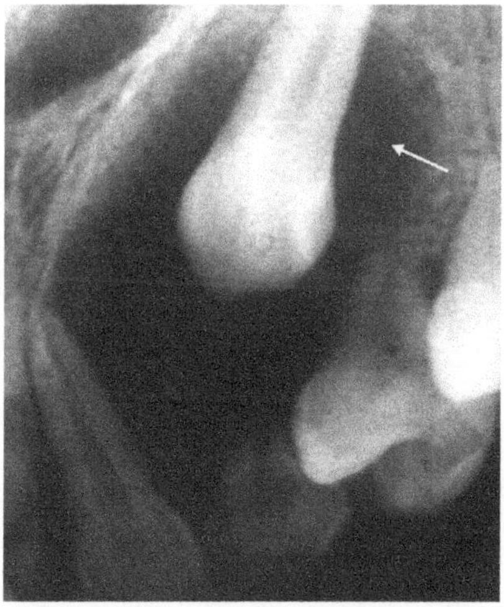

Fig. 17.6: Periapical radiograph of maxillary canine region shows radiolucent lesion with small foci of calcification (white arrow) along with impacted canine tooth

Differential diagnosis:
- Dentigerous cyst
- Ameloblastoma
- Ameloblastic fibroma
- Follicular cyst
- Gingival cyst
- Calcifying odontogenic cyst.

Odontogenic Myxoma

They are benign tumor arise from the mesenchymal portion of the (connective tissue) dental papilla, which produce either excessive fibrous collagen (fibroma) or excessive ground substance (myxoma).

Age: Young adults.

Frequency: Rare.

Site: Commonly involves premolar-molar areas of mandible and rarely zygomatic process of maxilla.

Size: Variable in size.

Shape:
- Multilocular
- Occasionally unilocular in early stages
- May be associated with a congenital missing or unerupted tooth.

Outline:
- Well-defined with corticated border
- Maxillary lesions are poorly defined.

Internal structure:
- Radiolucent with thin radiopaque septa or trabeculae.
- Small and uniform locules appear as a "*honey comb*" or "*soap bubble pattern*".
- Perpendicular type arrangements of trabeculae in the radiolucent described as a "*tennis-racket pattern*" (**Fig. 17.7**).

Effects:
- Displacement and loosening of adjacent teeth
- Root resorption is rare
- Buccal and lingual cortical plate expansion.

Differential diagnosis:
- Ameloblastoma
- Central giant cell granuloma
- Cherubism

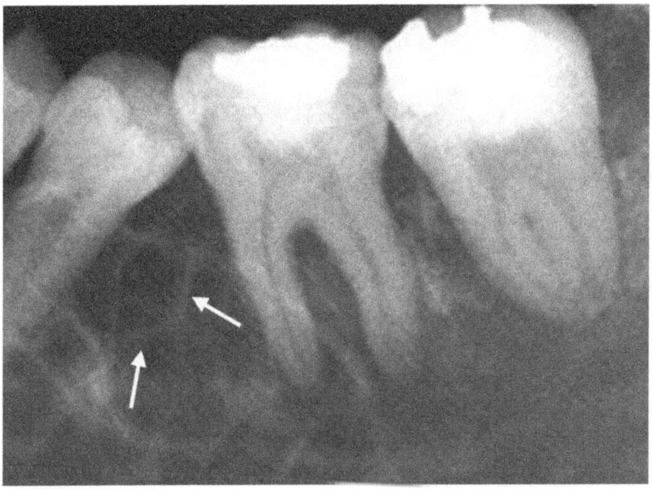

Fig. 17.7: Odontogenic myxoma in relation to lower premolar region shows multilocular with septa running at right angles to each other appears as tennis-racket (white arrows)

- Aneurysmal bone cyst
- Central hemangioma.

Odontoma

Odontoma is a benign tumor containing all the various component tissues of teeth. It is the most common odontogenic tumor, which results from a budding of extraodontogenic epithelial cells from the dental lamina. Some authors consider odontoma is a hamartoma rather than a neoplasm and refer to as odontogenic hamartoma.

Odontoma are grouped into two types:

1. Compound odontoma
2. Complex odontoma.

One more type of odontoma histologically as, ameloblastic fibro-odontoma.

Age: 2nd decade of life.

Frequency: Most common odontogenic tumor.

Site:

- Compound variety of odontoma occurs in the anterior maxilla in association with crown of an unerupted canine.

- Complex odontoma are found in the mandibular 1st and 2nd molar area.

Size: 1–3 cm in diameter.

Outline:
- Well-defined with smooth or irregular border.
- Corticated border.

Internal structure: The contents of these lesions are largely radiopaque.
- Compound odontoma have a number of teeth like radiopaque structures with in a well-defined borders **(Fig. 17.8A)**.
- Complex odontoma contain an irregular mass of calcified dental tissue bearing no resemblance in shape of a tooth appeared as completely radiopaque lesion with surrounded by radiolucent line **(Fig. 17.8B)**.

Effects:
- Odontoma are associated with impaction, malpositioning, malformation, diastema and devitalization of adjacent teeth.
- Expansion of the cortical plate observed in larger lesions.

Differential diagnosis:
- Cemento-ossifying fibroma
- Adenomatoid odontogenic tumor
- Periapical cemental dysplasia.

Nonodontogenic Tumors

Nonodontogenic tumors of the jaws are arising from the tissues other than odontogenic tissues, e.g. nervous tissue, fibrous tissue and cartilaginous tissue.

Benign intraosseous nonodontogenic tumors arise from the nervous tissue (nerve sheath and nerve fibers). These tumors commonly occur in the body and ramus of the mandible as the mandibular canal conveys a larger neurovascular bundle for a longer distance than any other bony canal in the body.

Nonodontogenic tumors can be grouped into:
- *Ectodermal nonodontogenic tumor:*
  - Neurilemmoma (schwannoma)
  - Traumatic neuroma
- *Mesodermal tumors:*
  - Osteoma
  - Central hemangioma
  - Arteriovenous fistula

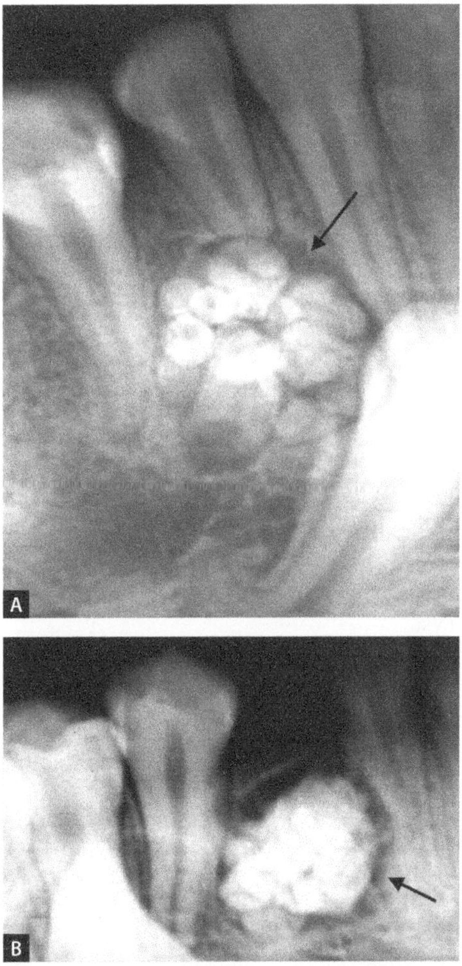

Figs 17.8A and B: Odontoma. (A) Compound odontoma; different tooth-like structures are seen with radiolucent margin; (B) Complex odontoma; calcified tooth structure arranged haphazardly within the radiolucent halo

  - Chondroma
  - Osteoblastoma
- *Mixed tumors:*
  - Neurofibroma
  - Neurofibromatosis (Von Recklinghausen's disease)

Neurilemmoma (Schwannoma)

It is the tumor of nerve tissue arising from the Schwann cells. It is most common in all neural tumors.

Age: 2nd and 3rd decade of life.

Frequency: Common nerve tumor.

Site: Posterior to the mental foramen of mandibular jaw.

Shape: Solitary or multilocular appearances.

Outline: Well-defined and cyst-like lesion with sclerotic border.

Internal structure: Round radiolucent areas of bone destruction. In that radiolucent different loculations or areas of cortical bone erosion appeared as a multilocular mimics the ameloblastoma.

Effects:
- Root resorption of adjacent teeth
- Jaw expansion
- Expansion of mandibular canal, mental foramen, mandibular foramen.

Differential diagnosis:
- Periapical cyst
- Ameloblastoma.

Neurofibroma

Benign well-circumscribed tumors caused by proliferation of Schwann cells in disorderly pattern.

Age: Young patient.

Frequency: Rare.

Site: Mandibular canal.

Shape:
- Usually appear unilocular
- Occasionally multilocular.

Outline: Sharply defined and corticated.

Internal structure:
- Well-defined unilocular radiolucent lesions.
- In some cases multilocular.

Effects: Enlargement of the canal.

Differential diagnosis: Vascular lesions.

Osteoma

It is a benign tumor arises from a cartilage or embryonal periosteum occurring in the skull and face. It is not clear that osteoma is a benign neoplasm or hamartoma. Structurally, osteoma can be grouped into three types:

1. Those composed of compact bone
2. Composed of cancellous bone
3. Composed of a combination of compact and cancellous bone.

Age: More than 40 years of age.

Frequency: Common among the bony neoplasm.

Site:

- Lingual side of the ramus
- Inferior mandibular border below the molars
- Condylar and coronoid process
- Frontal sinus.

Size: Small but some may become large enough to cause severe damage.

Outline: Well-defined borders.

Internal structure:

- Uniform radiopaque in compact bone.
- In cancellous bone, evidence of internal trabecular structure.

Effects: Displaced adjacent soft tissues such as muscles and cause dysfunction.

Differential diagnosis:

- Mature ossifying fibroma
- Early osteogenic sarcoma
- Chondroma
- Chondrosarcoma.

Central Hemangioma

It is a congenital anomaly in which proliferation of blood vessels leads to a mass that resembles a neoplasm. It occurs in the vertebrae and skull and rarely in the jaws.

Age: Young adults.

Frequency: Rare.

Site: More common in body and ramus of the mandible than maxilla.

Outline:
- In some cases lesion is well-defined and corticated
- Other cases it may be ill-defined.

Internal structure:
- It appeared as a radiolucent lesion with enlargement of trabecular spaces and the trabeculae are coarse, dense and well-defined suggestive of *"soap bubble"* **(Fig. 17.9)** or *"honey comb"* appearances.
- In some cases demonstrates the expanding lesion may show a "sunray" or "sunburst image".
- Occasionally, small areas of calcification found in a vein (phleboliths) within surrounding soft tissues.

Effects:
- Resorption of root.
- Entire length of mandibular canal is enlarged and appeared as a serpiginous path.
- Mandibular and mental foramen may be enlarged.

Differential diagnosis:
- Giant cell tumor
- Traumatic bone cyst
- Keratocyst.

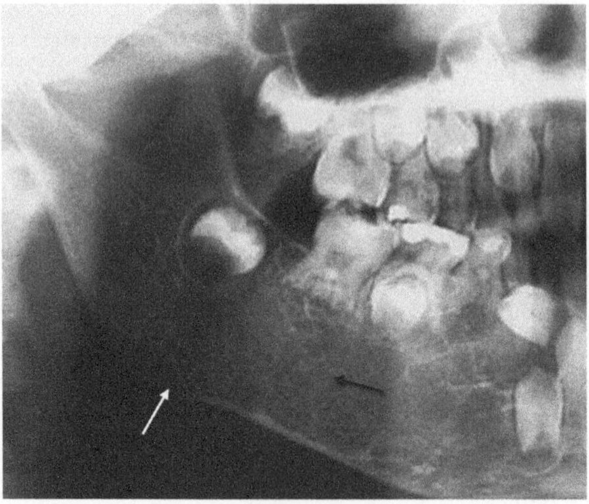

Fig. 17.9: Central hemangioma on cropped panoramic radiograph; thin and course trabeculae appears as soap bubble (black arrow) and thinning of cortex results in pathological fracture (white arrow)

MALIGNANT DISEASES OF THE JAW

Malignant tumors represent an uncontrolled growth of tissue. They are locally invasive and ability to metastasize regionally to lymph nodes or distantly to other sides.

Malignant tumors are growing by invasion and destruction of surrounding bone without cortical expansion and they spread rapidly, destroying bone leaving teeth in position and no evidence of root resorption.

Etiology: Malignancy may be mainly caused by:
- Viruses
- Prolonged exposure to radiation
- Genetic defects
- Exposure to carcinogenic chemical
- Tobacco.

Malignant diseases are classified based on histopathologically into:
- *Carcinomas* (lesions of epithelial origin)
- *Sarcomas* (lesions of mesenchymal origin)
- *Metastatic lesions* (lesions from distant sides).

Differences between carcinoma and sarcomatous lesions with examples are tabulated in **Table 17.2**.

Carcinoma

Squamous Cell Carcinoma

It is the most common malignant tumor of epithelial origin arising in the oral mucosa. It is characterized initially by invasion of malignant epithelial cells into the underlying connective tissue and spread into deeper soft tissues and adjacent bone, local regional lymph nodes and ultimately to distant sites such as lung, liver and kidney.

Clinically, squamous cell carcinoma appears initially as a white or red irregular patchy lesions of the epithelium into central ulceration, rolled or indurated border with regional lymphadenopathy as lesion advanced.

Age: Adults over 50 years.

Frequency: Rare, but the most common oral malignant tumor.

Site: Tumor commonly involves lateral border of the tongue invades into the posterior part of mandible. Lesions also found in the lip, floor of the mouth, attached gingiva, tonsils, soft palate and buccal vestibule but uncommon in hard palate.

Table 17.2: Difference between carcinoma and sarcoma

Features	*Carcinoma*	*Sarcoma*
Origin	Epithelial tissue	Connective tissue
Site	Cutaneous and lining mucosa	Cartilage (chondrosarcoma) Bone (osteosarcoma) Fat (liposarcoma) Muscle (leiomyosarcoma) Fibrous tissue (fibrosarcoma) Blood cells (Leukemia) Lymphoid tissue (Lymphosarcoma) Myeloid tissue (Myeloid sarcoma)
Age group	Usually over 50	Usually below 50
Frequency	Common (90% all cancer)	Rare (1% all cancer)
Behavior	Malignant	Malignant
Preferred route of metastasis	Lymph nodes	Blood borne
In situ phase	Yes	No
Growth rate	Rapid	Slower
Growth type	Infiltration and invasion. Spread throughout body through lymph node	"Ball-like" masses and tend to push adjacent structures. Spread by satellite nodules
Involvement of lymph node	Lymph node involvement is common	No involvement of lymph node
Response to chemotherapy	More	Less
Blood supply	Rich	Less
Most common site	Anywhere	Liver and lung
Surrounding area	No pseudocapsule, hence difficult to determine extent of lesion	Pseudocapsule surrounding the lesion

Carcinoma	*Sarcoma*
• Squamous cell carcinoma	• Osteosarcoma
• Primary intraosseous carcinoma	• Chondrosarcoma
• Mucoepidermoid carcinoma	• Fibrosarcoma
• Pleomorphic carcinoma	• Ewing's sarcoma
• Acinic cell carcinoma	• Leukemia
• Adenoid cystic carcinoma	• Malignant lymphoma
• Adenocarcinoma	• Burkitt's lymphoma Multiple myeloma

Size: Variable

Shape: Irregular area of bone destruction often appears as saucer shaped.

Outline: Irregular and mouth eaten, poorly defined, not corticated, finger-like projections.

Internal structure: Lesions shows complete radiolucent, occasionally small residual normal trabecular bones are visible within the radiolucency.

Effects: Adjacent teeth may be displaced and loosened, destruction of surrounding bone may result in pathological fracture.

Differential diagnosis: Osteomyelitis, osteoradionecrosis.

Primary Intraosseous Carcinoma

(Squamous cell carcinoma originating in bone, Intra-alveolar carcinoma, Intra-alveolar epidermoid carcinoma)

Primary intraosseous squamous cell carcinoma is defined as a type of squamous cell carcinoma arising within the jaws, having no connection with the oral mucosa and presumably developing from the residues of the odontogenic epithelium. It may arise within the jaws either from a previous odontogenic cyst or *de novo.*

WHO classified the lesion as odontogenic carcinoma. There are several classifications but Waldron and Mustoe's classification is widely accepted according to which, primary intraosseous squamous cell carcinoma may have different origins.

Type 1: PIOC exodontogenic cyst,

Type 2a: Malignant ameloblastoma,

Type 2b: Ameloblastic carcinoma arising *de novo*, ex ameloblastoma or ex-odontogenic cyst, *Type 3:* PIOC arising *de novo*, (a) Keratinizing type (b) nonkeratinizing type.

Type 4: Intraosseous mucoepidermoid carcinoma.

Primary intraosseous carcinoma (PIOC) arising *de novo* must be considered, if no cystic component of other odontogenic tumor cell is demonstrated.

To consider this lesion in the jaws as PIOC, it should meet three specific criteria:

1. Histological evidence of squamous cell carcinoma,
2. Absence of ulcer formation on the overlying mucosa, and

3. Absence of a distant primary tumor at the time of diagnosis and at least six months during the follow-up period.

Etiology of PIOC is not clear probably it arises from the remnants of odontogenic tissues, either the epithelial rests of Malassez or the remnants of dental lamina. The epithelial remnants proliferate and transform into odontogenic carcinoma, a process that is potentially triggered by an inflammatory process.

Age: 6–7th decades of life and more cases reported in men.

Frequency: Rare, but the most common carcinoma arising from the bone.

Site: Majority of the cases occur in the posterior mandible as painful non-ulcerated lesions.

Size: Variable

Shape: Unilocular radiolucency resembling cyst.

Outline: Irregular and poorly defined

Internal structure: A unilocular radiolucent without evidence of bone production **(Fig. 17.10)**.

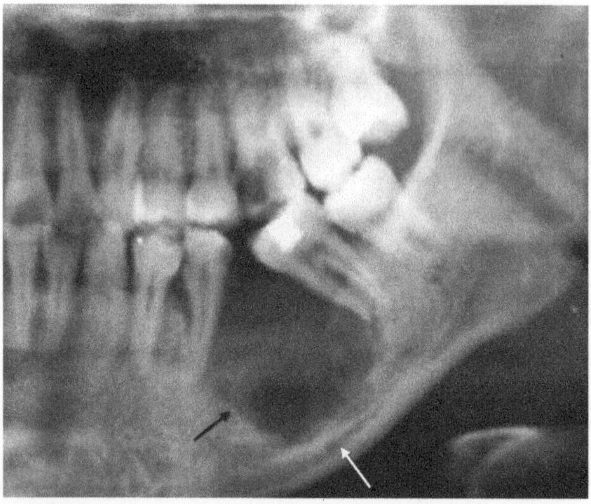

Fig. 17.10: Primary intraosseous carcinoma arising from the bone; a radiolucent without evidence of bone production and poorly defined border (black arrow). Note displacement of inferior alveolar canal (white arrow)

Effects:
- It does not cause root resorption or displacement.
- It tends to grow around obstructions such as teeth or other anatomical structures rather than displace them.
- It invades along the path of least resistance.

Differential diagnosis:
- Radicular cyst
- Ameloblastic carcinoma
- Clear cell odontogenic carcinoma
- Odontogenic ghost cell carcinoma
- Malignant variant of calcifying epithelial odontogenic tumor.

Sarcoma

Osteosarcoma

Osteosarcoma is a malignant tumor of bone.
There are three main types:
1. Osteolytic.
2. Osteosclerotic
3. Mixed lytic and sclerotic.

Age: Adults about 30 years old.

Frequency: Very rare, but the most common malignant tumor of bone.

Site: Posterior part of mandible including the tooth bearing region, angle and ramus of mandible.

Size: Variable.

Shape:
- Lesion is usually radiolucent with no peripheral sclerosis.
- If the lesion involves the periosteum, typical *"sun ray"* or *"sunburst"* spicules or *"hair-on-end"* appearances (if the lesion grows rapidly but steadily, the periosteum will not have enough time to lay down even a thin shell of bone, and the pattern may appear quite different. In such cases, the tiny fibers that connect the periosteum to the bone (Sharpey's fibers) become stretched out perpendicular to the bone. When these fibers ossify, they produce a pattern sometimes called "sunburst" or "hair-on-end" periosteal reaction, depending on how much of the bone is involved by the process **(Fig. 17.11A)**.
- If the periosteum is elevated and maintains its osteogenic bone called as *"Codman's triangle"* (A Codman triangle is not actually a full triangle. Instead it is often a pseudotriangle on radiographic

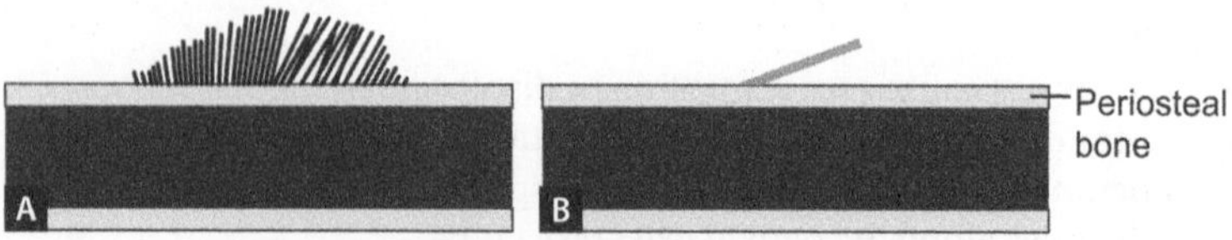

Figs 17.11A and B: Schematic representation of periosteal bone reactions. (A) Sunburst appearance; (B) Codman's triangle

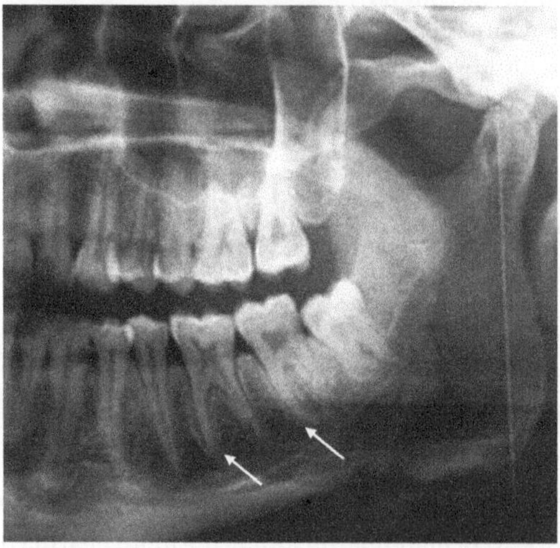

Fig. 17.12: Cropped panoramic radiograph shows osteosarcoma; note initial radiographical appearance of widening of periodontal ligament space on mandibular first and second molar (arrows)

findings with ossification on the original bone and one additional side of the triangle which forms a two-sided triangle with one open side. This two-sided appearance is generated due to a tumor (or growth) that is growing at a rate which is faster than the periosteum can grow or expand, so instead of dimpling, the periosteum tears away and provides ossification on the second edge of the triangle **(Fig. 17.11B)**. The most common causes of a Codman's triangle are *osteosarcoma, Ewing sarcoma and osteomyelitis.*

Internal structure:

Early features:

- Widening of periodontal ligament space **(Fig. 17.12)**.
- Poorly-defined radiolucent area around one or more teeth.

Later features:
Osteolytic lesion:
- Unilocular
- Ill-defined with moth-eaten outline
- Loosening of teeth.

Mixed lesion:
- Poorly defined radiolucent area with variable internal radiopacity
- Obliteration of normal trabecular pattern
- Expansion and perforation of the cortical margins
- Distortion of the alveolar ridge.

Effects:
- Antral or nasal cortical wall may be lost in maxillary lesions.
- Mandibular lesions destroy the cortex of the inferior alveolar nerve canal and lamina dura of the involved teeth.

Differential diagnosis:
- Fibrosarcoma
- Metastatic carcinoma
- Chondrosarcoma
- Ossifying fibroma
- Fibrous dysplasia.

Fibrosarcoma

Fibrosarcoma is a malignant neoplasm composed of fibroblast which fails to exhibit bone or osteoid formation. It arises either from periosteum or periodontal membrane.

Age: Fourth decade.

Frequency: Rare lesions.

Site: Premolar/molar regions of the mandible.

Size: Variable.

Shape: Saucer-like depression.

Outline:
- Ill-defined borders (Ragged)
- Noncorticated borders.

Internal structure:
- Complete radiolucent
- Occasionally reactive osseous bone formation within the radiolucent lesion.

Effects:
- Destruction of alveolar process, inferior border of the jaw and inferior alveolar canal in mandible.
- In maxilla floor of the maxillary sinus, nasal floor are destroyed.
- Root resorption.
- Displacement and loosening of involved teeth.
- Widening of periodontal ligament space.
- Appearance of "*Codman's triangle*" or "*sunray appearance*" when the lesion disrupts the periosteum.

Differential diagnosis:
- Metastatic carcinoma
- Multiple myeloma
- Intraosseous carcinoma
- Osteosarcoma
- Chondrosarcoma
- Ewing's sarcoma.

Multiple Myeloma

It is a malignant tumor of plasma cells and most common malignancy of bone in adults, single lesions are called plasmacytoma and multiple lesions are termed multiple myeloma.

In multiple myeloma, there is proliferation of abnormal plasma cells in the bone marrow which replace the normal bone marrow tissues.

Intraorally, it causes pain, swelling, hemorrhage, paresthesia, mobility and migration of teeth and occasionally pathological fracture of jaw occurs.

Age: 35–70 years with mean age 60 years.

Frequency: Rare but common malignant tumor of bone.

Site: More commonly seen in posterior body and ramus of mandible than maxilla.

Size: Variable.

Shape: Lesions appeared as a multiple typical *"punched-out"* radiolucency **(Figs 17.13A and B)** but some have oval or cystic shape.

Outline:
- Well-defined but not corticated
- No sign of bone reaction at the periphery
- Some lesions appear ragged and infiltrative.

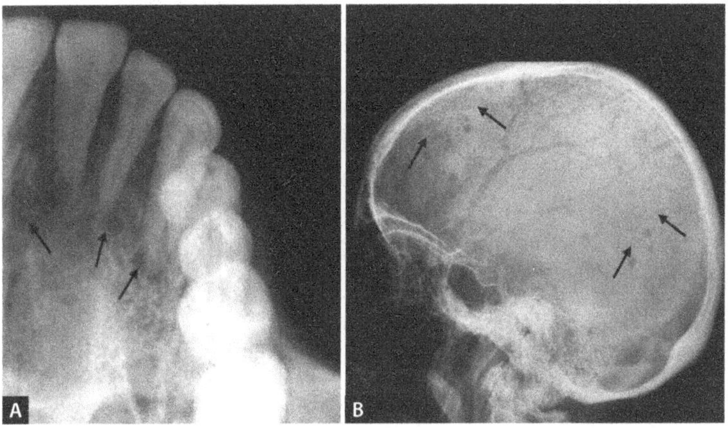

Figs 17.13A and B: Multiple myeloma; multiple punched out radiolucent. (A) Lesion on maxillary lateral occlusal view; (B) On lateral skull view

Internal structure: No internal structures are seen but occasionally islands of residual bone within the radiolucent lesions appeared as new trabecular pattern of bone.

Effects:
- Loss of lamina dura
- Cortical boundary lost in inferior alveolar canal in mandible
- Thinning of lower border of mandible.

Differential diagnosis:
- Metastatic carcinoma
- Osteomyelitis
- Brown's tumors of hyperparathyroidism.

Leukemia

Leukemia is a malignant tumor of hematopoietic stem cells in which abnormal proliferation of immature white blood cells occurs.
Leukemia is divided into two groups:
1. Acute leukemia
2. Chronic leukemia.

In *acute leukemia* primitive white blood cells are released into the blood but in *chronic leukemia* proliferation of abnormal cells which retain many of the morphological features of the normal cells.

Orally leukemia manifests as a gingival hyperplasia, profuse gingival bleeding, petechiae, loose teeth and ulceration.

Age:
- Acute leukemia occurs in children
- Chronic leukemia seen in older age people (50–70 years).

Site:
- Areas of developing teeth
- Localized around the periapical region of the tooth.

Size: Variable.

Shape: Patchy radiolucent areas, later it may coalesce to form larger areas of radiolucent region of bone.

Outline: Ill-defined.

Internal structure:
- Patchy areas of radiolucency
- Rarely foci of bone may be seen within these lesions.

Effects:
- Displacement of developing teeth
- Thinning or disappearance of lamina dura lost
- Cortical outlines of follicles get affected
- Loss of crestal alveolar bone
- Single layer of periosteal new bone formation.

Differential diagnosis:
- Neuroblastoma
- Lymphoma
- Rarefying osteitis
- Metabolic disorders.

Ewing's Sarcoma or Round Cell Sarcoma

Ewing's sarcoma is a malignant tumor originating in the bone marrow from the mesenchymal connective tissue. It occurs in the long bones and rarely in the jaws, orally it causes loose teeth, paresthesia, ulceration, displaced teeth and trismus.

Age: 2nd decade of life, mostly below 30 years.

Frequency: Rarely occurs in jaws.

Site: Posterior areas of both jaws.

Size: Variable.

Shape: Round or ovoid with solitary radiolucent lesions.

Outline:
- Poorly demarcated
- Not corticated
- Ragged borders.

Internal structure: Complete radiolucent with occasionally little bone formation within the lesions.

Effects:
- New periosteal bone formation appeared as a "Codman's triangle" or "sunray" or "hair-on-end"
- Lamina dura disappear
- Cortical outlines of mandibular canal, inferior border of mandible is lost.

Differential diagnosis:
- Osteomyelitis
- Eosinophilic granuloma
- Osteosarcoma
- Chondrosarcoma
- Fibrosarcoma.

Metastatic Tumors (Secondary Malignancy)

It is the most common malignant tumor of the skeleton resulting from metastasis of primary carcinoma from a distant site.

Jaw involvements of metastatic tumors are less than 1%. Metastasis may occur from breast, lungs, kidneys, prostate glands, testis, bladder, ovary and cervix.

Patient may complain of dental pain and paresthesia of the mandibular nerve. The teeth may become mobile and pathologic fracture of the jaw or hemorrhage from the tumor site occurred.

Age: 5th–7th decade of life.

Frequency: Rare.

Site: Mandible is more commonly involved than maxilla. In mandible premolar and molar region are the frequently affected.

Size: Variable.

Shape: Polymorphous in shape (multiple small radiolucent lesions).

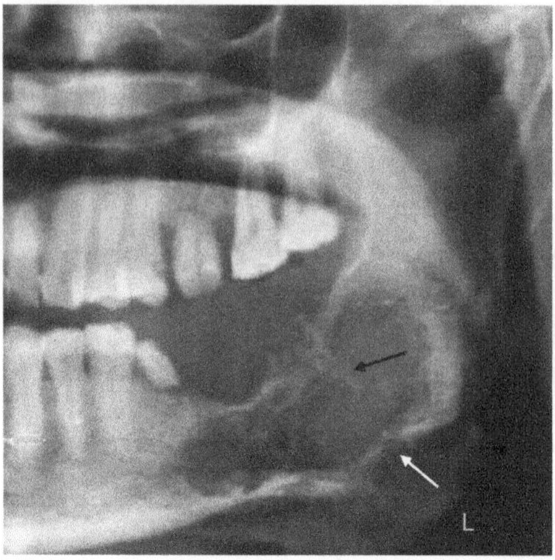

Fig. 17.14: Cropped panoramic radiograph revealed metastatic tumor; A radiolucent with well-defined border except on posterior region of the lesion. Residual trabeculae are shown (black arrow), thinning of the inferior border of mandible (white arrow)

Outline:
- Moderately well demarcated but no cortication or encapsulation at the margins
- Some have ill-defined margins.

Internal structure:
- Generally, lesions are radiolucent
- Some lesions shows residual trabecular bone within the radiolucent
- Multiple small radiolucent lesions with normal bone between the foci **(Fig. 17.14).**

Effects:
- Loss of lamina dura
- Enlarged periodontal ligament space
- Loss of supporting alveolar bone results in floating of teeth
- Destruction of cortical wall in mandibular canal, dental follicle, inferior border of mandible, sinus and nasal fossa.

Differential diagnosis:
- Multiple myeloma
- Squamous cell carcinoma.

CHAPTER

18

Fibro-osseous Lesions of the Jaw

Various diseases of bone that appear in the jaws develop from some disorders of one of the components of the osseous tissue. In most cases, the cause of the lesions of bone is unknown. Some of these, bone diseases are localized and manifest as a single lesion (e.g. simple bone cyst and giant cell granuloma, etc.), others may appear in multiple bones (e.g. fibrous dysplasia, Paget's disease, etc.) still others are systemic, affecting all bones (e.g. osteopetrosis).

Fibro-osseous lesions are the group of pathologic disturbances characterized by the replacement of the normal bone by a fibrous tissue composed of collagen fibers and fibroblasts containing various amount of calcified tissue.

Fibro-osseous lesions may vary from extensive and cosmetically disfiguring or functionally disturbing processes to small localized asymptomatic area that are discovered only in the course of a routine radiographic study.

Radiographically, these lesions appeared as a diffuse, ground glass and more well-defined cyst-like areas that may appear radiolucent or contain varying amount of radiopaque materials (mineralization).

Classification of Fibro-osseous Lesions

Based on origin of tissue, fibro-osseous lesions are classified into two types **(Table 18.1)**:

1. Periodontal membrane origin
2. Medullary bone origin

FIBROUS DYSPLASIA

This term was first suggested by *Lichtenstein* in 1938 as a designation for multiple (polyostotic) bone lesions.

Fibrous dysplasia characterized by proliferation of fibrous tissue and resorption of normal bone in localized area and subsequent replacement of varying amounts of abnormal-appearing bone.

Table 18.1: Classification of fibro-osseous lesions based on their origin of tissue

Origin	*Lesions*
1. Periodontal membrane	Cemento-ossifying fibroma Periapical cemental dysplasia (Cementoma) Florid cemento-osseous dysplasia (Gigantiform cementoma)
2. Medullary bone	Fibrous dysplasia Paget's disease Cherubism Aneurysmal bone cyst Giant cell tumor Hyperparathyroidism (Brown's tumor)

Fibrous dysplasia encompasses two clinical forms:

1. *Monostotic fibrous dysplasia:* Characterized by a single lesion affecting the jaws, particularly the posterior part of the maxilla.
2. *Polyostotic fibrous dysplasia:*
   a. *Jaffe type:* Multiple bone lesions, skin pigmentation (Café-au-lait spots) and hyperfunction of endocrine glands.
   b. *Albright syndrome:* More severe form of Jaffe type.

Patient with jaw involvement may complaint unilateral facial swelling or enlarging alveolar process. These lesions tend to be structurally weak and are, therefore, prone to pathologic fracture. Alkaline phosphatase may be elevated in up to 30% of patients with polyostotic fibrous dysplasia, and a dramatic rise may herald malignant degeneration. Malignant degeneration occurs in less than 1% of cases of fibrous dysplasia. Malignancies are almost exclusively osteosarcoma. For unknown reasons, monostotic and craniofacial lesions have the greatest potential for malignant degeneration. Pain, rapid growth of a lesion and a dramatic elevation of alkaline phosphatase may herald malignant transformation.

Age:

- Monostotic fibrous dysplasia occurs in older age group.
- Polyostotic fibrous dysplasia occurs in young children (Below 10 years).

Frequency: Rare, although monostotic type is more common (70%) than polyostotic type.

Site: Posterior part of maxilla.

Size: Variable.

Shape: Round and unilocular.

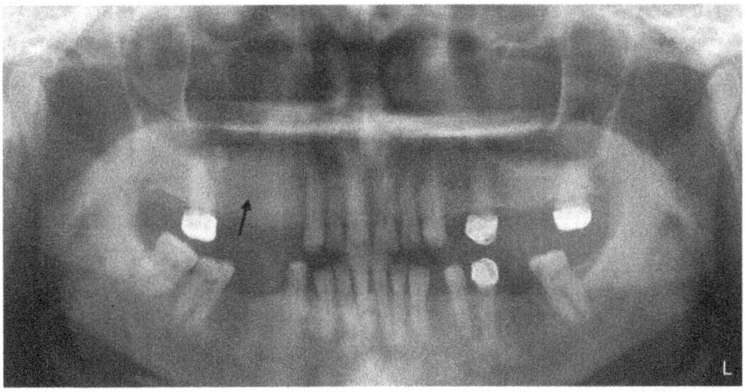

Fig. 18.1: Monostatic type of fibrous dysplasia in panoramic radiography shows short, thin and irregularly arranged trabecular pattern appears as a ground-glass pattern

Outline: Initially, lesions appear as well defined with corticated margins. As lesions mature, it becomes ill-defined and gradual merging with normal peripheral bone.

Internal structure: Initially, lesions shows radiolucent gradually to abnormal trabeculae are evident these trabeculae are shorter, thinner irregularly shaped this creates a radiopaque pattern produce typical *"Ground-glass" or "Orange*-peel" or "Co*tton*-wool" appearances **(Fig. 18.1)**.

Effects:
- Adjacent teeth often displaced.
- Loss of lamina dura
- Interfere with normal eruption of teeth
- Buccal and lingual cortical plate expansion
- Obliteration of the antrum
- Narrow periodontal ligament space.

Differential diagnosis:
- Hyperparathyroidism.
- Paget's disease.
- Periapical cemental dysplasia.
- Osteogenic sarcoma.
- Juvenile ossifying fibroma.

PAGET'S DISEASE (OSTEITIS DEFORMANS)

It is a condition of abnormal resorption and deposition of bone tissue in one or more bones. The disease may involve many bones simultaneously but it is not a generalized skeletal disease.

Typically, early stages of the disease are characterized by intense bone resorption (osteoclastic activity) resulting in irregularly-shaped resorption cavities. Later stages vigorous bone deposition (osteoblastic activity) leads to formation of woven bone.

Clinically, it manifests as a enlarged and deformed affected bone results in bowing of legs, enlargement of skull and jaws, separation and movement of teeth results in malocclusion. Dentures may be tight in edentulous patients.

Age: Middle and old age with peak age is 40 years.

Frequency: Rare.

Site: Maxilla is more common than mandible.

Size: Variable.

Internal structure: Generally, Paget's disease shows three radiographic stages:

1. Early radiolucent resorptive stage.
2. Granular or ground glass appearing.
3. Denser and more radiopaque stage.

Trabeculae are altered in number and shape.

- In early stage, they are less in number and they arranged in a horizontal linear pattern which is more common in the mandible.
- Trabeculae are short with random orientation and may have a granular pattern.
- Trabeculae may be arranged into rounded radiopaque patches of abnormal bone producing *"cotton-wool"* appearance **(Fig. 18.2)**.
- Overall density of the jaws may decrease.

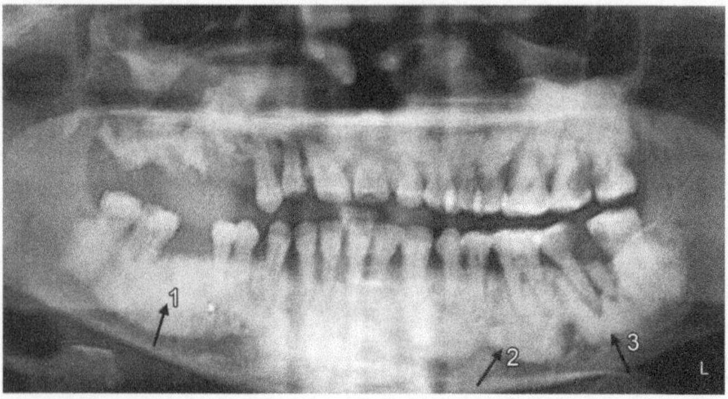

Fig. 18.2: Panoramic radiograph reveals fibrous dysplasia; Ground-glass or cotton-wool appears in right mandibular posterior region (1st arrow), dense radiopaque lesion seen on left mandibular posterior region (2nd and 3rd arrows)

Effects:

- Enlargement of affected bone like skull, jaws and sinus.
- Disappeared lamina dura.
- Hypercementosis develops on involved teeth, which is characteristic of Paget's disease.
- Teeth may be displaced.

Differential diagnosis: Florid-osseous dysplasia.

CHERUBISM

Cherubism is a rare, inherited developmental abnormality that causes bilateral enlargement of the jaws which produces cherubic facial appearance in the child.

Clinically, cherubism presents as a painless, firm, bilateral enlargement of the lower face, enlargement submandibular lymph nodes may occur.

Age: Early childhood between 2–6 years of age.

Frequency: Rare.

Site:

- Commonly in posterior part of mandible (Ramus of the mandible)
- Occasionally, it occurs in tuberosity of maxilla.

Size: Variable.

Shape:

- Multilocular.
- Symmetrical bilateral lesions.

Outline:

- Smooth.
- Well defined.
- Well corticated.

Internal structure: Radiolucent with internal radiopaque septa producing a multilocular appearance.

Effects:

- Expansion of buccal and lingual cortical plates
- Complete encroachment of maxillary lesions into the antrum
- Teeth are displaced, sometimes deciduous teeth exfoliated early.

Differential diagnosis:

- Giant cell granuloma
- Multiple odontogenic keratocyst.

ANEURYSMAL BONE CYST

Aneurysmal bone cyst is a reactive lesion of bone rather than a cyst or neoplasm. It represents an exaggerated, localized proliferative lesion of vascular tissue in bone containing giant cells.

Age: Under 30 years of age

Frequency: Rare

Site: Variable

Shape: Multilocular with round shape

Outline: Well defined

Internal structure: Radiolucent with evidence of faint internal trabeculation **(Fig. 18.3)**.

Effects:
- Adjacent teeth displaced and resorption of root.
- Buccal and lingual cortical plate expanded.

Differential diagnosis:
- Giant cell granuloma.
- Ameloblastoma.
- Cherubism.

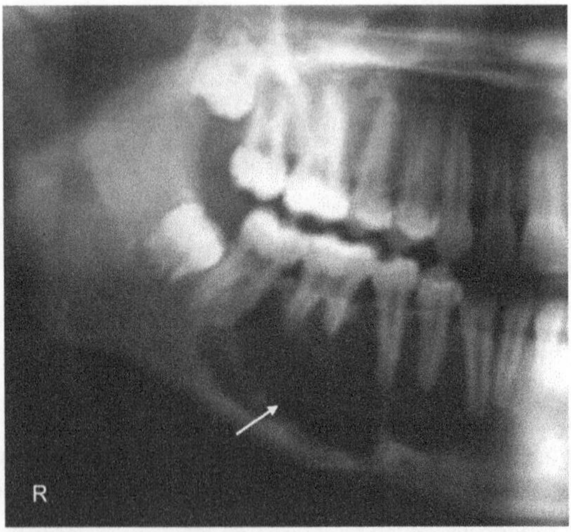

Fig. 18.3: Cropped panoramic radiograph shows aneurysmal bone cyst

CENTRAL GIANT CELL GRANULOMA

Central giant cell granuloma is a reactive lesion of bone. It manifest as a painless swelling and affected bone get tender on palpation.

Age: Young adults below 20 years of age.

Frequency: Rare.

Site:

- More in mandible, epicenter is anterior to the first molar. Sometimes, it crosses the midline.
- In maxilla, it occurs anterior to the cuspid region.

Size: Variable

Shape: Multilocular

Outline: Well-defined and well-corticated

Internal structure: Radiolucent larger lesions have thin internal septa producing the multilocular or sometime *"honeycomb"* appearance.

Effects:

- Adjacent teeth displaced and resorption.
- Buccal and lingual cortical plate expanded and perforation **(Fig. 18.4)**.

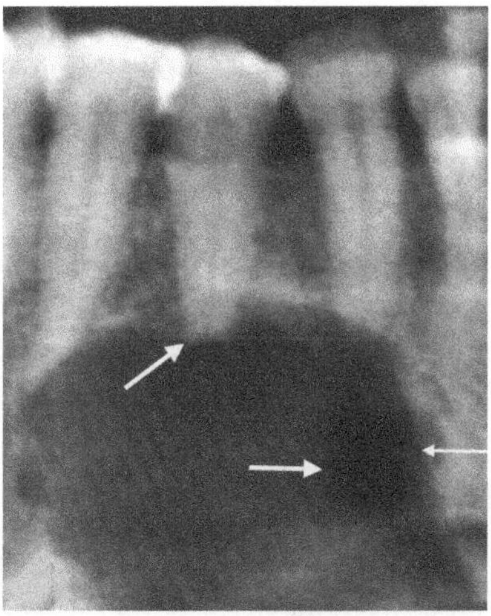

Fig. 18.4: Periapical radiograph demonstrates central giant cell granuloma; note resorption of root (arrows) and perforation of cortical plate

Differential diagnosis:
- Ameloblastoma.
- Odontogenic myxoma.
- Aneurysmal bone cyst.
- Brown tumors of hyperparathyroidism.

BROWN TUMORS OF HYPERPARATHYROIDISM

Primary hyperparathyroidism caused by either hyperplasia or an adenoma of the parathyroid or secondary hyperparathyroidism caused by kidney disease result in increased secretion of parathromone. This cause generalized skeletal bone resorption leading to osteopenia (Generalized decrease in bone density) bone pain or pathological fracture and raises the plasma-calcium levels. Localized cyst-like giant cell lesions (Brown tumors) can also develop in the jaws and long bones. Hence, the term osteitis fibrosa cystica applied to this condition.

Radiographically, it appears as:
- Osteopenia in the skull vault producing a fine overall stippled pattern to the bone, hence the description *"pepper pot"* skull.
- In the jaws, osteopenia producing a very fine trabecular pattern often described as *"ground glass"*.
- Loss of lamina dura surrounding all the teeth and thinning or loss of normal thick cortical bone of the lower border of the mandible **(Fig. 18.5)**.
- Localized radiolucent cyst-like giant cell lesions termed Brown tumors.

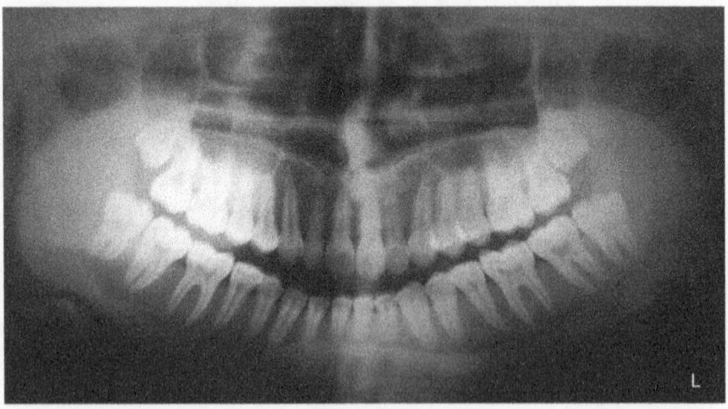

Fig. 18.5: Panoramic radiograph revealed hyperparathyroidism; note very fine trabecular pattern appeared as ground glass, generalized loss of lamina dura and loss of cortical bone of the lower border of the mandible

PERIAPICAL CEMENTAL DYSPLASIA OR CEMENTOMA

It is a localized change in normal bone metabolism that results in the replacement of the normal cancellous bone components with fibrous tissue and cementum-like material.

Clinically, the involved teeth are vital and no history of pain or sensitivity and the lesion located near the apex of the tooth.

Age: Middle age with mean age is 39 years.

Frequency: Rare

Site: Variable

Shape: Irregularly shaped or round or oval-shaped over the apex of the tooth.

Outline: Well-defined and radiolucent border.

Internal structure: Internal structure varies depending on the maturity of the lesion.

In early stage: Normal bone resorbed and replaced with fibrous tissue appeared radiographically as a radiolucency at the apex of the involved tooth **(Fig. 18.6A)**.

In mixed stage: Radiopaque tissue (cementum or abnormal bone) appears in the radiolucent structure **(Fig. 18.6B)**.

In mature stage: Internal aspect may be completely radiopaque and thin radiolucent margins can be seen at the periphery.

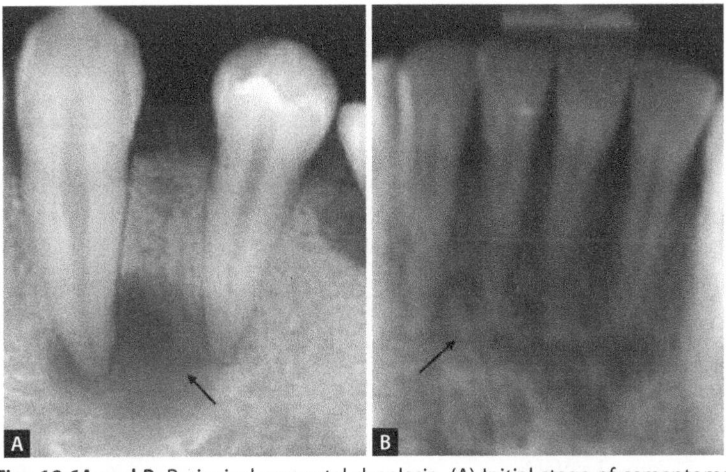

Figs 18.6A and B: Periapical cemental dysplasia. (A) Initial stage of cementoma appears as radiolucent lesions with absence of pulpal or periodontal infections; (B) Mixed or intermediate stage, where radiopaque lesions surrounded by radiolucent halo

Effects:
- Normal lamina dura of the teeth involved is lost.
- Widen periodontal ligament space.
- Occasionally, some root resorption may occur.
- Elevate the floor of the antrum.

Differential diagnosis:
- Periapical infections.
- Benign cementoblastoma.
- Odontoma.

CEMENTO-OSSIFYING FIBROMA

It consists of highly cellular, fibrous tissue that contains varying amounts of abnormal bone or cementum-like tissue. In the past, this lesion was classified as two different entities as a cementifying fibroma and ossifying fibroma depending on whether bone or cementum was the predominant calcified product.

When the cementum is the predominant calcified tissue the term cementifying fibroma, if bone is the calcified tissue called as ossifying fibroma.

Age: Young adults.

Frequency: Rare apical region.

Site:
- Premolar/molar regions of mandible above the inferior alveolar canal.
- In maxilla, it occurs in the canine fossa and zygomatic arch area.

Size: Variable.

Outline: Well-defined thin radiolucent line represents a fibrous capsule surrounding the bone.

Internal structure: Mixed radiolucent—radiopaque density lesions that produce more cementum like material may contain solid radiopacity (cementicles).

Effects:
- Displacement of teeth and inferior alveolar canal.
- Expansion of outer cortical plates of bone.
- Missing lamina dura.
- Resorption of teeth may occur.

Differential diagnosis:
- Fibrous dysplasia.
- Juvenile ossifying fibroma.
- Calcifying odontogenic cyst and tumors.
- Adenomatoid odontogenic tumors.

Appendices

APPENDIX 1

LIST OF RADIOGRAPHIC DESCRIPTIONS
(in Alphabetical Order)

Radiographic description	Conditions
1. Ball-in-hand appearance	Benign salivary gland tumors
2. Balloon-like appearance	Follicular cysts Aneurysmal bone cyst
3. Candle-stick appearance	Pyknodysostosis Progressive systemic sclerosis
4. Chalk-like appearance	Osteopetrosis (marble bone disease) Hyperparathyroidism Pyknodysostosis
5. Cherry blossom pattern	Sialography of Sjögren's syndrome
6. Codman's triangle	Osteosarcoma
7. Cotton-wool appearance	Paget's disease Odontogenic fibroma Fibrous dysplasia of bone
8. Eggshell appearance	Ameloblastoma Multilocular cyst
9. Filling defect	Salivary grand tumor
10. Floating-teeth appearance	Histiocytosis-X Squamous cell carcinoma of the gingiva Papillon-Lefèvre syndrome Advanced periodontitis
11. Ghost teeth appearance	Regional odontodysplasia
12. Ground-glass appearance	Fibrous dysplasia of bone Ossifying fibroma Osteosarcoma
13. Hair-on-end appearance	Thalassemia Sickle cell anemia Central hemangioma Paget's disease
14. Heart-shaped radiolucency	Nasopalatine cyst
15. Honeycomb appearance	Ameloblastoma Central hemangioma

16. Moth-eaten appearance	Squamous cell carcinoma of the gingiva Malignant lymphoma Chronic osteomyelitis
17. Mottled appearance	Fibrous dysplasia of bone Ossifying fibroma
18. Onion-peel (skin) appearance	chronic osteomyelitis Eosinophilic granuloma Ewing's sarcoma
19. Pear-shaped appearance	Globulomaxillary cyst Radicular cyst
20. Pencil-line appearance	Ameloblastoma Traumatic bone cyst Calcifying epithelial odontogenic cyst (Gorlin's cyst)
21. Pressure-type appearance	Squamous cell carcinoma of the gingiva
22. Punched-out appearance	Multiple myeloma Histiocytosis-X
23. Rootless teeth	Dentin dysplasia
24. Sand-like appearance	Adenoameloblastoma Calcifying epithelial odontogenic cyst (Gorlin's cysts) Calcifying epithelial odontogenic tumor (Pindborg tumor)
25. Salt and pepper appearance	Hyperparathyroidism Traumatic bone cyst Aneurysmal bone cyst Giant cell granuloma
26. Scalloping pattern (margins)	Dentigerous cyst Traumatic bone cyst Aneurysmal bone cyst Giant cell tumor
27. Soap bubble appearance	Ameloblastoma Giant cell granuloma Central hemangioma
28. Spiked root	Malignant histiocytoma Burkitt's lymphoma
29. Sunray (burst) appearance	Osteosarcoma Metastatic carcinoma Ewing's sarcoma

30. Tennis racket appearance — Odontogenic myxoma
31. Worm-eaten appearance — Carcinoma of the gingiva; Malignant lymphoma; Chronic osteomyelitis

Soap-bubble appearance refers to circular cyst-like radiolucency of various sizes; whereas Honey-comb appearance refers to much smaller circular cyst-like radiolucency of even sizes.

Moth-eaten appearance and worm-eaten appearance are used interchangeably.

APPENDIX 2

LAMINA DURA

Lamina dura is a radiographic feature appears as a thin radiopaque line surrounding the roots of the teeth, which represents the alveolar bone proper.

Presence of intact lamina dura around the apex of the tooth strongly suggestive of vital pulp. Absence of lamina dura indicates either periapical pathology or occasionally improper angulation of the X-ray beam.

Absence of lamina dura can be classified into:

- Localized
- Generalized
- Miscellaneous

Localized Absence of Lamina Dura

- Periapical periodontitis
- Periapical abscess
- Periapical granuloma
- Periapical cyst condensing osteitis
- Periodontal abscess
- Osteomyelitis

Generalized Absence of Lamina Dura

- Hyperparathyroidism
- Osteomalacia
- Fibrous dysplasia
- Rickets
- Leukemia

- Multiple myeloma
- Paget's disease
- Osteopetrosis
- Osteoporosis
- Hyperphosphatasia
- Systemic sclerosis
- Metastatic tumor
- Cushing's syndrome
- Hypoparathyroidism
- Acromegaly
- Hypervitaminosis D

Thick Lamina Dura

- Osteopetrosis
- Scleroderma

APPENDIX 3

CEMENTUM

Absence of Cementum

- Cleidocranial dysplasia
- Hypophosphatasia

Hypercementosis

- Acromegaly
- Paget's disease

APPENDIX 4

CLASSIFICATION OF RADIATION

Based on Ionization

- *Ionizing radiations:*
  i. Alpha rays
  ii. Gamma rays
  iii. X-rays
  iv. Cosmic waves

- *Nonionizing radiations:*
  i. Beta rays
  ii. Cathode rays
  iii. Ultraviolet rays
  iv. Infrared rays
  v. Microwaves
  vi. Radiowaves

Based on Utilization

- *Therapeutic:*
  i. Beta rays
  ii. Infrared waves
  iii. Ultraviolet waves
  iv. X-rays
- *Non-therapeutic/diagnostic:*
  i. X rays
  ii. Ultrasound waves
  iii. Magnetic waves

Based upon Nature of Radiation

- *Particulate:*
  i. Alpha rays
  ii. Beta rays
  iii. Cathode rays
- *Electromagnetic:*
  i. Radiowaves
  ii. Microwaves
  iii. Infrared waves
  iv. Ultraviolet rays
  v. X-rays
  vi. γ-rays

APPENDIX 5

BONY LESIONS OF THE JAWS

Bony lesions of the jaws are classified into:

- Radiolucent
  - Unilocular
  - Multilocular
- Radiopaque

Unilocular Radiolucent Lesions

- Periapical abscess
- Periapical granuloma
- Periapical cyst
- Periapical scar
- Surgical defect
- Osteomyelitis
- Dentigerous cyst
- Early stage of cementoma
- Periodontal abscess
- Traumatic bone cyst
- Unilocular ameloblastoma
- Aneurysmal bone cyst
- Central giant cell granuloma
- Brown tumor of hyperparathyroidism
- Early stage of odontoma
- Submandibular gland depression
- Incisive canal cyst
- Midpalatine cyst
- Median mandibular cyst
- Malignant tumor
- Residual cyst

Multilocular Radiolucency

- Ameloblastoma
- Central giant cell granuloma
- Giant cell lesion of hyperparathyroidism
- Cherubism
- Odontogenic myxoma
- Odontogenic keratocyst
- Aneurysmal bone cyst
- Metastatic tumor
- Central hemangioma
- Calcifying epithelial odontogenic tumor
- Chondroma
- Fibrous dysplasia
- Osteomyelitis
- Adenomatoid odontogenic tumor
- Paget's disease

Radiopaque Lesions

- Condensing osteitis or chronic focal sclerosing osteomyelitis
- Periapical idiopathic osteosclerosis
- Periapical cemento-osseous dysplasia
- Foreign bodies
- Hypercementosis
- Later stage of cementoma
- Later stage of odontoma
- Later stage of osteoblastoma
- Osteogenic sarcoma
- Advance stage of Paget's disease
- Maxillary or mandibular tori
- Calcifying odontogenic cyst
- Cemento-ossifying fibroma
- Chondroma and chondrosarcoma
- Exostosis
- Sialolith
- Rhinolith
- Antrolith
- Phleboliths

APPENDIX 6

BENIGN AND MALIGNANT LESIONS OF THE MANDIBLE

Cystic Lesions

- Periapical (radicular) cyst
- Follicular (dentigerous) cyst
- Odontogenic keratocyst (OKC)
- Primordial cyst
- Residual cyst
- Solitary bone cyst (traumatic, simple, hemorrhagic bone cyst)
- Medullary pseudocyst
- Aneurysmal bone cyst
- Static bone cavity (Stafne cyst [not a true cyst])

Solid Lesions

Benign

- *Odontogenic:*
  - Odontoma
  - Ameloblastoma
  - Odontogenic myxoma
  - Calcifying epithelial odontogenic tumor (Pindborg tumor)
  - Cementoblastoma
  - Ameloblastic fibroma
  - Adenomatoid odontogenic tumor
- *Nonodontogenic*
  - *Osseous lesions:*
    - Ossifying fibroma
    - Juvenile-ossifying fibroma
    - Periapical cemental dysplasia
    - Florid cemento-osseous dysplasia
    - Exostosis (torus mandibularis)
    - Osteoma
    - Fibrous dysplasia
    - Paget's disease
  - *Nonosseous lesions:*
    - Neurofibroma
    - Schwannoma
    - Central giant cell granuloma (giant cell reparative cyst)
    - Arteriovenous malformation (AVM)
    - Central hemangioma
    - Epulis fissuratum

Malignant

- *Odontogenic:*
  - Odontogenic carcinoma (ameloblastic carcinoma, primary intraosseous carcinoma, etc.)
  - Odontogenic sarcoma (ameloblastic fibrosarcoma, ameloblastic fibro-odontosarcoma, etc.)
  - Odontogenic carcinosarcoma
- *Nonodontogenic:*
  - Osteosarcoma
  - Chondrosarcoma
  - Metastasis
  - Fibrosarcoma

- Leiomyosarcoma
- Malignant lymphoma
- Leukemia
- Multiple myeloma and plasmacytoma
- Squamous cell carcinoma

Metabolic Bone Lesions

- Osteoporosis
- Osteomalacia
- Renal osteodystrophy
- Osteitis fibrosa cystic

APPENDIX 7

MANDIBULAR LESIONS BY LOCATION

Anterior Mandible

- Adenomatoid odontogenic tumor
- Periapical cemental dysplasia
- Florid cemento-osseous dysplasia
- Central giant cell granuloma
- Odontoma

Posterior Mandible

- Follicular (dentigerous) cyst
- Odontogenic keratocyst
- Solitary bone cyst (traumatic, simple, hemorrhagic bone cyst)
- Ameloblastoma
- Calcifying epithelial odontogenic tumor (Pindborg tumor)
- Cementoblastoma
- Ossifying fibroma
- Ameloblastic fibroma
- Ameloblastic carcinoma
- Metastasis
- Arteriovenous malformation
- Static bone cavity (Stafne cyst [not a true cyst])
- Odontogenic myxoma

Nonspecific Location

- Periapical (radicular) cyst
- Metabolic

APPENDIX 8

MAXILLOFACIAL BONY LESIONS BY ORIGIN OF TISSUE

Origin of tissue	*Benign tumor*	*Malignant tumor*
Osteogenic	• Osteoma • Osteoid osteoma • Osteoblastoma	Osteosarcoma
Chondrogenic	• Chondroblastoma • Chondromyxoid fibroma • Chondroma • Osteochondroma	Chondrosarcoma
Fibrogenic	Fibrous dysplasia	Fibrosarcoma
Vascular	Hemangioma	Hemangioendothelioma
Hematopoietic		• Plasmacytoma • Lymphoma
Others	• Gaint cell tumor • Aneurysmal bone cyst • Meningioma	• Chordoma • Ewing's sarcoma

APPENDIX 9

ADVANCED IMAGING TECHNIQUES

Ionizing Radiographic Techniques

- Stereoscopy
- Xero-radiography
- Digital radiography
- *Contrast radiography:*
  - Sialography
  - Pulpography
  - Arthrography
  - Angiography
  - Lymphography
  - Urography
  - Barium swallow, meal and enema
  - Enhanced or contrast computed tomography
  - Enhanced or contrast magnetic resonance imaging

- *Tomography:*
  - Simple tomography
  - Emission tomography
  - Computed tomography
  - Cone beam computer tomography (CBCT)
- *Nuclear medicine:*
  - Scintigraphy
  - Positron emission tomography (PET)
  - Single photon emission computed tomography (SPECT)

Nonionizing Radiation Techniques

- Ultrasonography
- Magnetic resonance imaging
- Thermography

APPENDIX 10

SITE SPECIFIC JAW LESIONS

- *Anterior mandible:*
  - Lateral periodontal cyst
  - Glandular odontogenic cyst
  - Calcifying epithelial odontogenic cyst
  - Periapical cemental dysplasia
  - Central giant cell granuloma
- *Posterior mandible:*
  - Dentigerous cyst
  - Buccal bifurcation cyst
  - Odontogenic keratocyst
  - Lateral periodontal cyst
  - Traumatic bone cyst
  - Ameloblastoma
  - Calcifying epithelial odontogenic tumor
  - Complex odontome
  - Ameloblastic fibroma
  - Odontogenic myxoma
  - Benign cementoblastoma
  - Central odontogenic fibroma
  - Neurilemmoma
  - Osteoma
  - Central hemangioma

- Cemento-ossifying fibroma
- Central giant cell granuloma
- Aneurysmal bone cyst
- Langerhans cell histiocytosis

- *Ramus:*
  - Traumatic bone cyst
  - Ameloblastoma
  - Osteoma
  - Central hemangioma
  - Aneurysmal bone cyst
  - Cherubism
- *Anterior maxilla:*
  - Radicular cyst
  - Glandular odontogenic cyst
  - Calcifying cystic odontogenic tumor
  - Nasopalatine duct or incisive canal cyst
  - Paget's disease
  - Compound odontome
  - Adenomatoid odontogenic tumor
  - Central giant cell granuloma
- *Posterior maxilla:*
  - Fibrous dysplasia
  - Paget's disease
- *Above the mandibular canal:*
  - Odontogenic tumors
  - Odontogenic cysts
  - Osteomyelitis of jaws
- *Below the mandibular canal:*
  - Fibrous dysplasia
  - Traumatic bone cyst
  - Stafnes cyst
  - Nonodontogenic tumors

APPENDIX 11

CLASSIFICATION OF LESIONS ACCORDING TO THE GROWTH PATTERN

- *Lesions with anteroposterior extension:*
  - Odontogenic keratocyst
  - Traumatic bone cyst
  - Odontogenic myxoma

- *Lesions with mediolateral extension:*
  - Radicular cyst
  - Residual cyst
  - Dentigerous cyst
  - Ameloblastoma
  - Calcifying epithelial odontogenic tumor
  - Odontomas
  - Ameloblastic fibroma
  - Adenomatoid odontogenic tumor
  - Benign cementoblastoma
  - Osteoblastoma

APPENDIX 12

RADIOGRAPHIC APPEARANCE OF MAXILLARY SINUS IN DISEASE

- *Completely radiopaque:*
  - Maxillary sinusitis
  - Retention pseudocyst/antral pseudocyst
  - Mucocele
  - Papilloma
  - Osteoma
  - Squamous cell carcinoma
  - Odontogenic cysts
  - Fibrous dysplasia
- *Partially radiopaque:*
  - Antral polyps
  - Antrolith
  - Odontogenic tumors
  - Dental structure displaced into the maxillary sinus

APPENDIX 13

DISEASES ASSOCIATED WITH WIDENED PERIODONTAL LIGAMENT SPACE

- Progressive systemic sclerosis (Scleroderma)
- Chondrosarcoma
- Osteosarcoma
- Osteogenic sarcoma

- Acute periapical abscess
- Periodontal infections associated with local factors
- Periodontal infections associated with systemic diseases
  - Diabetes mellitus
  - Acquired immunodeficiency syndrome (AIDS)

APPENDIX 14

RADIOGRAPHIC FAULTS

Radiographic errors	*Causes*	*Solutions*
Light radiograph:		
• *Processing errors:*	• Underdeveloped (temperature too low/time too short/thermometer inaccurate) • Depleted developer solution • Diluted or contaminated developer • Excessive fixation	• Regularly check and maintain the temperature of the developer and fixer. • Proper follow the time temperature chart and adjust the developing and fixing time. • Replenisher added to depleted or diluted developer.
• *Exposure errors:*	• Insufficient mA • Insufficient kVp • Insufficient exposure time • Film-source distance too great • Film placed reversed in mouth	• Proper selection of mA, kVp and exposure time. • Maintain film-source distance 8 inch in bisecting and 12–16 inch in paralleling technique, but in extraoral radiography, pre-adjusted distance is facilitated. • Check the side of film towards X-ray source.
Dark radiograph		
• *Processing errors:*	• Overdeveloped (temperature too high/time too long) • Developer concentration too high • Inadequate fixation • Accidental exposure to light • Improper safe lighting	• Regularly check and maintain the temperature of the developer and fixer. • Proper follow the time temperature chart. • Light proof darkroom. • Use GBX filter with 15 watts orange color bulb. Maintain working area distance 4 feet from the safe light. • Perform penny test to check the stray light.

Contd...

Contd...

Radiographic errors	*Causes*	*Solutions*
• *Exposure errors:*	• Excess mA • Excess kVp • Excess exposure time • Film source distance too short	• Proper selection of mA, kVp and exposure time. • Maintain film-source distance 8 inch in bisecting and 12–16 inch in paralleling technique.
Insufficient contrast (Low contrast)	• Underdevelopment • Underexposure • Insufficient kVp • Excessive film fog	• Proper follow the time temperature chart and adjust the developing and fixing time. • Proper selection of kVp. • High kVp reduces the film fog.
Film fog	• Improper safelight (improper filter; excessive bulb wattage; inadequate distance between safelight and work surface; prolonged exposure to safelight). • Light leaks (cracked safelight filter; light from doors, vents, or other sources). • Overdevelopment • Contaminated solution • Deteriorated film (stored at high temperature; stored at high humidity; exposed to radiation; outdated).	• Light proof darkroom. • Use GBX filter with 15 watts orange color bulb. Maintain working area distance 4 feet from the safe light. • Perform penny test to check the stray light. • Adjust the developing time. • Avoid contamination of processing solution. • Use lead film storage box to avoid accidental exposure.
Dark spots or lines	• Fingerprint contamination • Film contaminated with developer before processing. • Excessive bending of films during exposure. • Film in contact with tank or another film during fixation	• Always hold the film at the edges. • Working area should be clean and free from developer solution. • Avoid excessive bending film during radiography. • Use film hangers during processing to avoid contact between each film.
Light spots	• Film contaminated with fixer before processing. • Film in contact with tank or another film during development.	• Working area should be clean and free from developer solution. • Avoid marking with pen or sharp items on the unexposed film.

Contd...

Contd...

Radiographic errors	*Causes*	*Solutions*
		• Use film hangers during processing to avoid contact between each film.
Yellow or brown stains	• Depleted developer • Depleted fixer • Insufficient washing • Contaminated solution	• Replenisher added to depleted or diluted developer.
		• Wash film in running water sufficiently to remove residual fixer. • Replace the aged processing solution.
Blurring	• Movement of patient • Movement of X-ray tube head • Double exposure	• Stabilize the patient and X-ray source during radiography. • Keep separately exposed with unexposed films.
Partial images (Cone cut)	• Partially immersed film in the processing solution. • Misalignment of X-ray tube head. • Improper film positioned during radiography.	• Completely immerse the film in the processing solution. • Proper position the tube head and the film.
Scratched film	Emulsion peeled off from the film.	Handle the film carefully.

APPENDIX 15

DISTRIBUTION OF JAW LESIONS BASED ON AGE

	Jaw lesions	*Age*
Jaw cysts	Dentigerous cyst	20–40 years
	Odontogenic keratocyst	2nd–3rd decades
	Calcifying epithelial cyst	10–19 years
	Incisive canal or nasopalatine cyst	40–60 years
Odontogenic jaw tumors	Ameloblastoma	40 years
	COT	Middle age
	AOT	5–50 years
	Odontogenic myxoma	Young adults
	Odontoma	Second decade

Contd...

Contd...

	Jaw lesions	*Age*
Nonodontogenic jaw tumors	Neurilemmoma	2nd–3rd decades
	Neurofibroma	Young age
	Osteoma	40 years
	Central hemangioma	Young adults
Fibro-osseous lesions	Fibrous dysplasia	Old age
	Paget's disease	40 years
	Cherubism	2–6 years
	Aneurysmal bone cyst	Less than 30 years
	Central gaint cell tumor	Less than 20 years
	Cementoma	Middle age
	Cemento-ossifying fibroma	Young adults
Malignant lesions	Squamous cell carcinoma	More than 50 years
	Osteosarcoma	30 years
	Fibrosarcoma	4th decade
	Multiple myeloma	30–70 years
	Leukemia	Children (Acute) Old age (Chronic)
	Ewing's sarcoma	Less than 30 years
	Metastatic tumor	5th to 7th decades

Index

Page numbers followed by *f* refer to figure, and *t* refer to table

D

E

F

G

K

L

M

N

O

P

Q

R

S